ONE STEP AHEAD OF OSTEOARTHRITIS

Stay flexible and keep moving

ONE STEP AHEAD OF OSTEOARTHRITIS

Stay flexible and keep moving

FRANCES IVE

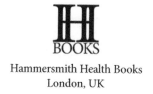

Hammersmith Health Books
London, UK

First published in 2019 by Hammersmith Health Books – an imprint of
Hammersmith Books Limited
4/4A Bloomsbury Square, London WC1A 2RP, UK
www.hammersmithbooks.co.uk

The information contained in this book is for educational purposes only. It is
the result of the study and the experience of the author. Whilst the information
and advice offered are believed to be true and accurate at the time of going to
press, neither the author nor the publisher can accept any legal responsibility or
liability for any errors or omissions that may have been made or for any adverse
effects which may occur as a result of following the recommendations given
herein. Always consult a qualified medical practitioner if you have any concerns
regarding your health.

British Library Cataloguing in Publication Data: A CIP record of this book is
available from the British Library.

Print ISBN 978-1-78161-164-7
Ebook ISBN 978-1-78161-165-4

Commissioning editor: Georgina Bentliff
Edited by: Carolyn White
Designed and typeset by: Julie Bennett of Bespoke Publishing Ltd.
Cover design by: Madeline Meckiffe
Cover image: © Jerry Lin/Shutterstock
Illustrations on pages 32-34, 44 and 48 by TechSet Ltd.
Index: Dr Laurence Errington
Production: Helen Whitehorn, Path Projects
Printed and bound by: TJ International, Padstow, Cornwall, UK

Contents

Foreword 1

As a GP I can prescribe thousands of pounds a year of NHS drugs or Consultant time for the treatment of arthritis. I cannot prescribe this book on the NHS, yet the advice it gives is absolutely critical to minimising the pain and suffering of osteoarthritis. I would go further and suggest in many cases it offers far more than I or my medical colleagues can. Keep in mind the ineffectiveness of many of the painkillers and other drugs used in osteoarthritis, the overuse of opioid painkillers such as morphine and tramadol, and indeed their addictive qualities and a raft of serious side-effects.

In 2018, an article in the *British Medical Journal*[1] stated: 'A recent systematic review focusing on adverse drug events in ambulatory care (in A and E) found prevalence rates ranging from 2.8% to 34.7% up to a quarter of which were judged preventable.' Another systematic review reported that 9.9% of all hospital admissions in people aged 65 years or over were as a result of an adverse drug event.

You must also add to this the growing evidence of poor diet, obesity and inactivity being among the causes of life-threatening and -shortening diseases.

The NHS has stated on many occasions that every 10 days of bed rest in hospital is the equivalent of 10 years of muscle ageing when it occurs in people over the age of 80, and it can take far longer to recover and a lot of hard work to get back to their previous condition.

A further study shows that inactivity increases early death by 7% and avoiding obesity could reduce deaths by nearly 4%.[2] Many academics, such as Sir Muir Gray, say, 'Sitting down is the new smoking'.

Many of us will face long-term illnesses, such as osteoarthritis, later in life. This book is not just about length of life, it is about something much more important – a happy and healthy life, whatever is thrown at you. It is about self-motivation and well-being. It should be prescribed on the NHS by all doctors. It can't be, but if you have osteoarthritis or want to live a happier and healthier life, buying this book is the best investment you could ever make.

Professor Sir Sam Everington, GP in Tower Hamlets, Chair of NHS Tower Hamlets Clinical Commissioning Group and a board member of NHS Clinical Commissioners

References

1.   Perez T, Moriarty F, Wallace E, McDowell R, et al. Prevalence of potentially inappropriate prescribing in older people in primary care and its association with hospital admissions: longitudinal study. *British Medical Journal* 2018; 363: k4524. Doi: https://doi.org/10.1136/bmj.k4524

2.   Ekelund U, Ward HA, Norat T, Luan J, et al. Physical activity and all-cause mortality across levels of overall and abdominal adiposity in European men and women: the European Prospective Investigation into Cancer and Nutrition Study (EPIC). *American Journal of Clinical Nutrition* 2015; 101(3): 613-621. Doi: 1, https://doi.org/10.3945/ajcn.114.100065

Foreword 2

This easy-to-read book offers sufferers of osteoarthritis new ways of managing their symptoms, which in turn leads to a more positive outlook on their prognosis.

So often people with a diagnosis of arthritis are given a life sentence of pain and misery. They are led to believe that nothing can be done and they must learn to live with the consequences of their disease. Frances offers hope and, without preaching, she offers tools that can be used to alleviate symptoms. She shows that by taking responsibility for our own health, improvements can be made.

Suggestions range from diet and lifestyle to alternative therapies and supplements. In fact, there are so many suggestions that no-one could fail to find areas where they can make changes and take charge.

I too suffer from osteoarthritis in my knee after years of sporting injuries but I am quite mobile and not in pain. I manage my symptoms with exercise, massage and diet and know that without these interventions I would not feel as good as I do.

Enjoy this book and the hope and inspiration it brings with it.

Barbara Cousins, nutritionist and author of *Easy, Tasty, Healthy* and the *Cooking Without* series

Acknowledgements

I would like to thank all the following who have helped me with certain aspects of this book:

Dr Christopher J. Etheridge; Dr Roger Wolman; Dr Rod Hughes; Professor Sir Sam Everington; Dr Tom Margham; Barbara Cousins; Dr Susan Aldridge; Dr Chris Steele; Versus Arthritis; British Acupuncture Council; Margaret Hills Clinic; Richard Kravetz; Ian O'Donnell; and Dr Miriam Ferrer of *Future You*.

I would like to thank the following for the use of their illustrations:
- Knee and hip exercise diagrams courtesy of Versus Arthritis www.versusarthritis.org.uk (pages 23-31)
- 'Get Paid While Running' (page 89) courtesy of Varidesk[†]
- 'How Much Pressure Are Your Hands Under?'(page 91) courtesy of Penclic

[†]Footnote: The citations for the Varidesk infographic are:
[*]Dr John Buckley (University of Chester). 'Standing-based office work shows encouraging signs of attenuating post-prandial glycaemic excursion.' 2013
[**]Harvard Medical School. Calories burned in 30 minutes for people of three different weights.
[***]Calories burnt during a marathon. NY Daily News (statistics from the Cleveland Clinic Center for Consumer Health Information)

About the author

Frances Ive has been a health journalist for more than 20 years, with over 100 articles published in national newspapers and consumer women's and health magazines. She runs the website www.healthysoul.co.uk, is a member of the Guild of Health Writers and has written several non-fiction books. Following the advice outlined in this book she has reduced pain and inflammation in her osteoarthritis and is able to manage it well.

Introduction

This book is about staying ahead of osteoarthritis, not letting it take you over; about staying mobile and, above all, enjoying life. It aims to make you feel much better.

It is for people who have early signs of osteoarthritis or have mild to moderate symptoms. But many of the tips could help someone with chronic arthritis and hopefully relieve inflammation and pain.

Whenever a doctor tells me that there is nothing they can do for a health problem, I decide to find out for myself what I can do. And so it was with osteoarthritis, which I had diagnosed in my hands and knee five years ago. With my experience as a health journalist and general interest in self-help and complementary medicine I tried to do everything I could to help myself, with considerable success.

I arrived on holiday in Devon a few years ago and could hardly get out of the car because I felt so stiff after the long journey. My knees and hands were painful and my whole body was aching. I decided to start with some changes to my diet – taking out certain foods and concentrating on trying to avoid acidic foods and drinks and making my intake more alkaline. I started taking supplements specific to osteoarthritis, and spent the week's holiday doing lots of swimming and going in the sauna.

Back at home I began doing exercises designed to help osteoarthritis, including using an exercise bike; I continued to play tennis, and attend yoga and tai chi classes, and had regular acupuncture treatments. At the time of writing this book my fingers have become much straighter than they were and my knee barely hurts when I play two hours of tennis.

I have not cured my osteoarthritis, but I am certainly managing it, and preventing it getting any worse. I do have pain when the weather changes and my thumbs react when I overuse them, but in general I live a normal, active life and hope to continue doing so in the future.

A word of warning – if you're buying this book for someone else who is resistant to change, they have to want to work on improving their condition!

Top tips for managing osteoarthritis

- **Keep your weight under control**: Being overweight puts huge strain on hips, knees and ankles, while shedding it can considerably reduce pain. Rheumatologists, who are specialists in arthritis, often recommend patients lose weight and do exercise. This can mean avoiding surgery, replacement joints and/or strong drugs. (See Chapter 2.)
- **Exercise regularly**: This is to strengthen muscles around joints and protect them, and to remain active and healthy. There are many types of exercise that help – cycling, swimming, and special physio exercises can help. You need to exercise according to your own flexibility and pain, but the more you remain active in your everyday life the better it is for your overall health. Of course, the knock-on effect of exercise is weight loss. (See Chapters 3 and 4.)
- **Food**: Some foods are acidic and can be bad for osteoarthritis, but alkaline foods are generally better for health. You can try to cut out foods that are very acidic (such as tomatoes) or eat them in moderation if you usually consume them on a daily basis. (See Chapters 5 and 6.)
- **Posture**: Review how you use your body – What position do you spend your day in? Are you sitting at a computer? How do you sleep at night? These issues are addressed in Chapters 9 and 10.
- **Footwear**: Shoes that absorb shock, such as trainers and running shoes, are the best to wear to protect hips, knees

and ankles. If you wear high heels you put enormous strain on your hips and knees.

- **Avoid walking down**: Going down steep hills or long staircases should be avoided if you already have arthritis in your knees. If you find you have to walk down a steep hill, try walking from side to side in a downwards zigzag to cut down the gradient. Take lifts rather than walking down too many stairs.

Chapter 1

Good health and osteoarthritis

The Spanish have a saying: *'La esperanza es lo ultimo que se pierde'* which means 'Hope is the last thing you lose'. Everyone needs hope in their lives and taking action to manage osteoarthritis is a positive move.

The aim of this book is to provide a range of helpful ways to manage osteoarthritis, and it can be used like a pick-and-mix to enable you to choose what type of exercise suits you, what changes you can make to your lifestyle and diet, and what practical measures or therapies you want to try.

Taking responsibility for your health

We know so much more about healthy living these days, and doctors, nutritionists, complementary therapists and, consequently, many other people have a much better idea about how to maintain and enhance our wellbeing.

In an attempt to modernise the NHS and promote good health, British people are being asked to take more responsibility for their own health. The advent of social prescribing in doctors' surgeries can only be seen as positive. It means that when someone visits their doctor with a variety of ailments, they will of course be treated if there is an obvious infection or serious illness, but doctors will try to establish the person's wellbeing and see if there are ways of improving their quality of life as well as the health problems they are taking to the GP.

It's quite common to think that good health means not being diagnosed with a serious illness. But what does it really mean? To attain and maintain good health we need to pay attention to several key aspects of our lives.

- **Sleep**: Everyone knows when they are getting good quality sleep for enough hours each night because they feel good and in control. If we're regularly getting short, interrupted nights we will start to feel depressed and anxious and any health problems are likely to become much worse.
- **Healthy food**: Making time to eat and enjoy three meals a day with plenty of vegetables and a good spread of nutrients sustains the body and keeps us feeling fit both mentally and physically. The digestive system accounts for some 70 per cent of the health of our immune system.
- **Mobility**: Most of us spend years taking our unimpeded mobility for granted, but it takes considerable effort to ensure that this continues as we get older. Inactivity leads to loss of muscle tone and strength, which are necessary to protect and support the joints. Conversely, activity and exercise stop us stiffening up and becoming immobile. Becoming immobile limits lives and can lead to isolation and subsequent emotional problems.
- **Relaxation**: For many people, life is so hectic that there is virtually no time to sit down and just be. Stress is a massive problem in this fast-moving technological age and it not only makes health issues worse but can actually cause them. Relaxing and having some quiet time are essential to keeping sane even if it's just for 10 minutes a day, as well as enjoying social activities or hobbies we love. Read about mindfulness and relaxation techniques in Chapter 11.
- **Environment**: Everyone needs to feel that they have

a home where their heart is, where they can relax and feel safe and comfortable. It means not contending with difficult neighbours, a dangerous area and/or pollution that is damaging to health. Think about how your environment affects you and, if it has a negative impact, find out about how you can change it.

A diagnosis of osteoarthritis

You go to the doctor with persistent pain or swelling in your joints and you may have an X-ray or an MRI scan. The diagnosis is osteoarthritis. So, what happens next? Provided you are not in chronic pain, you may be told that this is a normal part of the ageing process, and if you're lucky the doctor will give you some lifestyle tips.

At this point you have to take the bull by the horns and find out how you can maintain your mobility and prevent chronic inflammation and pain. Taking charge and managing your osteoarthritis are really the key to a hopeful future.

There's no magic bullet for curing osteoarthritis but it can be managed, enabling people who have it to remain active and enjoy a good quality of life through self-help: diet, weight loss, exercise, therapies, and a whole raft of practical measures. The overall aim is to remain mobile and pretty much pain-free, to continue enjoying an active and sociable life and not to suffer alone in silence.

'Focus on what is important to you in life – that is what you want to continue being able to do and what activities are special for you,' is the helpful advice given by Professor Sir Sam Everington, OBE (a GP in east London; Chair of NHS Tower Hamlets Clinical Commissioning Group; and NHS England's national adviser on general practice care models).

What is osteoarthritis?

Severe osteoarthritis is at best uncomfortable but at worst it is disabling and even crippling. Although it is often considered an inevitable part of ageing, there is much that can be done to prevent it getting severe. This book focuses on **osteo**arthritis, and only refers to **rheumatoid** arthritis to explain the difference.

The difference between rheumatoid arthritis and osteoarthritis

- Rheumatoid arthritis is an auto-immune disease, which means that the immune system attacks the body. Rheumatoid arthritis causes swelling, pain and stiffness in the joints, and it is managed with drugs when caught early.
- Osteoarthritis happens when there is a loss of cartilage – the protective surface over the ends of bones – particularly on the fingers, knees, toes, hips, base of thumb and spine. This can be seen and felt in some joints which are enlarged or swollen.
- There are several other types of arthritis which are less common, including psoriatic arthritis.

Osteoarthritis is the most common type of arthritis; it is thought to affect 8.75 million people in the UK. However, there are many other people who have aches and pains but have not been given a diagnosis, so the number could be much higher. It takes years to develop, so there is plenty of time to start being proactive.

Over time, cartilage, the protective surface over the end of the bones, wears away, and joints become swollen and painful. When it becomes severe there is so little cartilage that where the ends of bones meet (at the joints) they rub on each other and the joint may change shape.

In the case of the knee, the muscles surrounding the joint

become weaker and thinner, so exercise for the knees is very important because stronger muscles protect the knee joint (see Chapter 3, page 23).

Swollen and painful joints not only impede mobility, but arthritic fingers make it difficult to do things we expect to do all the time – such as opening bottles, picking things up, carrying shopping, and numerous other activities that we do with our fingers. Fortunately, there is plenty that can be done to alleviate pain and discomfort.

Statistics about osteoarthritis

It can start at around 40 years old, or even earlier, and the majority of older people have some osteoarthritis.

- Around 10 million people in the UK have arthritis, but the vast majority of these (8.75 million+) have osteoarthritis.[1]
- Fewer than 500,000 have rheumatoid arthritis.[2]
- Osteoarthritis affects all ages, but the majority of people with the condition (41 per cent) are over 65.[1]
- One third of over 45-year-olds have sought treatment for osteoarthritis – more women than men.[1]
- Between 1990 and 2010, disability due to osteoarthritis in the UK increased by 16 per cent.[3]

How osteoarthritis is diagnosed

Osteoarthritis can be found in the fingers and thumb joints, back, hips, knees, and toes. It is most common in the knees and hips, which are weight-bearing joints. Excessive use of a joint can lead to the cartilage being worn down. People who have overused their fingers, particularly with keyboards (especially the old manual typewriters), mobile phones, and other technological gadgets, may be more prone to it, as are sports people like footballers and tennis players, who have a tendency towards osteoarthritis in the knee.

It is also hereditary so if your mother or father has/had osteoarthritis, you are more likely to follow suit. If you have swollen or enlarged joints in your fingers, or your knee hurts when you walk up and down stairs or hills, the chances are you have early signs of osteoarthritis. Doctors can recognise it in the hands, but if it is not obvious they refer patients for X-rays and/or MRI scans. Sometimes an X-ray doesn't show up osteoarthritis, but an MRI scan shows it clearly.

Can you get better?

How often have you seen old men or women whose fingers are bent and gnarled, who can hardly walk or get outside? When you have the first few twinges of arthritis in your fingers or knees it doesn't mean that you will end up like them, but it's essential to take action to prevent it getting much worse. Even people with crippling arthritis might gain some relief from trying self-help approaches.

In the first stages of osteoarthritis doctors are unlikely to prescribe drugs. They may offer some lifestyle advice on exercise and suggest that you stay active. So, if you have been told, 'You just have to live with it', you don't have to!

Pain management

Living with constant pain is wearing and debilitating. It can affect sleep, make you depressed, and has other mental effects such as confusion and forgetfulness. It is a natural reaction not to want to move too much for fear of increasing the pain. Yet being immobile does not make you better in the long term, because you are likely to gain weight, and your muscles become weaker.

Long-term pain can make you so tired that daily activities become a chore and in some cases relationships become strained. All these problems have a negative effect on emotions as well, and it's not unusual for people who feel that they are losing their independence and mobility to become depressed (see Chapter 11).

Professor Sir Sam Everington emphasises that pain is contextual: 'If someone is in a warm cosy environment with their family the pain appears to be less.' Alternatively, if they are living alone and feeling less mobile, they are likely to become lonely and focus much more on their pain.

It has recently been assessed that 25 per cent of the population are lonely, but when they visit the GP, they present a long list of physical and mental problems, including insomnia, digestive pain and discomfort, back pain, anxiety, depression and many more ailments.

It is a fact that people who are enjoying their lives are less likely to focus on their ailments, and this is true of osteoarthritis too. There is plenty that can be done to alleviate the symptoms of arthritis – the inflammation and pain – rather than prescribing painkillers.

How is osteoarthritis treated?

So, what happens when you suspect that your finger joints are getting bigger and are painful or when your knee hurts as you go up and downstairs? In the past you would have been told to rest, but that advice has completely changed. In the US there is a serious addiction problem to opioid painkillers, with many people dying each year from this. In the UK, opiate drugs for osteoarthritis are not widely prescribed, because of the addiction problems in the US. No-one wants to become addicted to painkillers, nor do they want to become immobile and subsequently crippled.

Doctors usually advise taking painkillers such as paracetamol and codeine and NSAIDs (non-steroidal anti-inflammatory drugs), like ibuprofen, instead, and in some cases steroids. If this isn't working, doctors have the option to refer patients to a rheumatologist and/or a physiotherapist.

Dr Rod Hughes, a rheumatologist at St Peter's Hospital, Chertsey, Surrey, says: 'We see patients when the GP can no longer manage their pain, or because they cannot take anti-inflammatory drugs, due to intolerance or stomach problems.

'We have a wider range of drugs to use, including steroids which can be taken as tablets or injected into the joint or muscle. I'm a great fan of steroids, but they are very sensitive drugs that must be used carefully, because in large doses they can cause side-effects. In the right doses they are very effective.'

Easing the pain

Sometimes the pain is not actually felt in the joint but is in the muscles around the joint. They may be so tight and painful that the impact is felt around the area, so it's difficult to know where the pain is actually coming from. Massaging and exercising the muscles is worth doing routinely each day – after a bath, when you get up, after you've been sitting for a while.

There are many ways of soothing and relieving pain aside from medication, which are outlined in this book, and these include:
- Therapies such as chiropractic, osteopathy, acupuncture and massage (see Chapter 8).
- Hydrotherapy (often on the NHS) (see Chapter 3).
- Devices such as TENS (transcutaneous electrical nerve stimulation), ultrasound and laser (see Chapter 10).
- Alexander technique for releasing muscle tension (see Chapter 4).
- Herbal remedies (see Chapter 7).
- Bathing in warm water, especially with Epsom salts.
- Specific exercises (see Chapter 3).
- Heat – a hot water bottle, heated wheat or lavender pad, applied to the area.

- Cold – ice packs, a cold-water compress or even a pack of frozen peas applied to an inflamed and painful joint can ease the swelling and pain.
- Some people find magnet therapy helpful and you can buy bracelets and other jewellery containing magnets, and sometimes combining it with copper. Copper bracelets have been used for years for people with rheumatic conditions like osteoarthritis. Anecdotally, a lot of women claim that their gold wedding rings have kept that finger free from arthritis, whereas the other fingers may be swollen and deformed.
- Massage – massaging your hands with a base oil (almond oil, for instance) or cream can warm them and help ease pain. You could either put essential oil of ginger or cut up pieces of fresh ginger in oil and massage in – ginger is very warming. There are many oils available in a health food store that are good for tight muscles and painful joints.

Read on, this book is all about easing pain and inflammation!

Hip and knee replacements

The National Joint Registry[4] statistics show that in 2017 there were 105,306 hip and 112,836 knee replacement procedures performed on the NHS (in England, Wales and Northern Ireland), and there are additional procedures carried out in the private sector. In 98 per cent of cases of knee replacements, osteoarthritis is the cause, while for hip replacements 90 per cent of cases are due to osteoarthritis. The majority of operations are for women.

Dr Rod Hughes explains, 'There doesn't seem to be uniform agreement among surgeons about indications for surgery, but the degree of pain may well be the main reason. If a patient has tried physiotherapy, lost weight, and the tablets and injections are still failing, then surgery could be the answer, but there has to be X-ray evidence as well of course. Whenever a joint still has life in it, we try to keep it going.'

Hip replacements have been so successful that Dr Tom Margham, a GP in Tower Hamlets, and former Arthritis Research UK's primary care lead, points out that they are 'the most effective interventions in all of healthcare'. He says, 'For the right person at the right time of their life, they can really improve their quality of life. Not everyone benefits, but after 10 years, 90 per cent of replacement hips are still good, and 80 per cent are effective after 15.'

He continues, 'Hip replacements are more likely to stay in place than those in knees or other joints. Knees are inherently less stable and functional. There is often so much muscle wastage around the joint that they require a lot of prehabilitation prior to the operation and rehabilitation afterwards.'

There have sometimes been problems with the body reacting badly to the metal in replacement hips or knees or even causing infection. This could be due to allergies to certain metals, or because the patient already had some metal implants in the body.

Dr Margham explains, 'Some people do experience problems with the metal in replacement joints releasing ions and causing strong reactions in the body. There is a move now towards ceramic sockets with a metal stem and ball.'

Arthroscopies for knees

Dr Margham explains that arthroscopies (where the knee joint is flushed with saline) are less likely to be recommended now. 'These have been discredited as not having any effect, and the only reason a knee arthroscopy would be offered now is if a bit of cartilage had broken off and was causing a blockage'.

The effect of diet and exercise

Traditionally osteoarthritis has been thought to be due to wear and tear on the joints and this is a very plausible explanation. However, researchers at the University of Surrey have found that there is a link between metabolism and osteoarthritis.[5] This led them to state that osteoarthritis can potentially be prevented with a good diet and regular exercise.

'For too long osteoarthritis has been known as the "wear and tear disease",' according to the lead author of the review, Professor Ali Mobasheri, professor of musculoskeletal physiology, University of Surrey. He continues, 'It is important never to underestimate the significance of a healthy diet and lifestyle as not only do they impact upon our general wellbeing, but can alter the metabolic behaviour of cells, tissues and organs leading to serious illnesses.'

In their book *The Infection Game*, Dr Sarah Myhill and Craig Robinson claim[6] that osteoarthritis is mostly due to an allergy to a virus, foods and/or microbes from the fermenting gut which spill over into the bloodstream with the potential to drive inflammatory reactions at other sites, such as the joints, especially where there has been damage in the past. They point out that this is worsened if the body is too acidic (see Chapter 6, Food and drink – acid or alkaline?).

There has been some research which indicates that osteoarthritis could be an inflammatory disease,[7] but this is not conclusive yet. As with many health issues, research findings are changing the picture all the time.

Chapter 2

Looking at weight loss

Over half of adults in the UK (62 per cent) are either overweight or obese, according to a report from Arthritis Research (now Versus Arthritis).[1] Weight loss is one of the most written and talked about subjects in the media. New diets emerge all the time encouraging people to shed those pounds and enjoy a better life.

With osteoarthritis there is a very valid reason for losing weight – it makes sense that the heavier you are, the more pressure you put on your weight-bearing joints, especially the knees and hips. But the good news is that you can avoid surgery and even the need for drugs if you lose some weight.

Dr Roger Wolman, consultant rheumatologist at the Royal National Orthopaedic Hospital, says that exercise, weight loss and wearing the right shoes can keep a patient off drugs and injections and prevent surgery. He cites a woman who was due to have a knee replacement. 'She lost 10 kilos (1 stone 8 lb) and the pain improved so much that she was able to come off the waiting list for surgery. If someone commits to weight loss the reduction in pain is significant.'

Facing reality

Weight is a very delicate subject and people don't really like talking about it. Friends and family may avoid bringing up the subject for fear of causing upset but in reality, it is one of the most important, indeed vital, things that can be done to improve health. Some doctors sometimes prefer not to tackle the subject, as no-one wants to be criticised. However, rheumatologists and other doctors can feel duty bound to encourage a patient to lose weight if they feel that it would ease the pain and inflammation of osteoarthritis.

Professor Sir Sam Everington feels that doctors need to suggest losing weight in a caring way. He tells patients that it might help them and the reason that he's telling them is because he wants to help them, but that he is not judging them. Not everyone will have such an understanding doctor of course.

The right time

Sometimes it is helpful to be told by a doctor that you need to lose weight for the sake of your health because it can provide the momentum needed to get started. It's important to be in the right state of mind and have an attitude that you will succeed. Depending on how much weight you need to lose, it can affect you emotionally as well as physically. If you have been overweight or obese for much of your life, there are mental challenges to overcome as well when embarking on weight control. Sometimes people gain weight because of emotional problems that date back to childhood and the way our parents dealt with issues around eating. It's very important, therefore, to get some emotional support when starting a slimming regime, and there are organisations that can help with this. For someone who has a huge amount of weight to lose, it is advisable to seek medical advice to monitor progress.

Take it slowly

What can be daunting is thinking about the total amount of weight that needs to be lost. If you need to lose, say, five stone, it sounds such a lot that it can be off-putting. Having smaller goals makes it much more manageable and easier to cope with – starting with increments of 3.18 kg (half a stone/7 lb), for instance. When you achieve this, you are more likely to feel empowered to carry on and lose some more.

Few people find losing weight easy, but it brings such benefits that it is good to find a way of eating healthily that suits you, cut portions down at mealtimes and avoid fattening snacks. It doesn't matter what your age is, you can still benefit from shedding some pounds, provided you need to.

The rewards are good – you start to feel better; people remark on how good you look, and you may become more active. Fitting into that pair of trousers that have been waiting hopefully in the wardrobe is a great incentive. In short, losing pounds can have far-reaching and positive effects in many ways, not just physically, and can give back a quality of life that has been all but forgotten.

Chapter 5 explains which food types are necessary to eat to be healthy and lose weight. What you eat plays a major part in losing weight, but it is important to exercise, which doesn't necessarily mean joining a gym and pumping iron.

For those who are not used to exercise, it's important to start slowly. Taking the stairs instead of the lift is a good start (provided this doesn't make your knees feel worse!). Gentle walking instead of taking the car or public transport can make you fitter and help with the ultimate goal of losing weight (see Chapter 3).

Putting pressure on the joints

It is obvious that the more weight a joint has to support the more pressure it is under and this can lead to (and aggravate) osteoarthritis in the knees, hips and feet. Someone who is overweight or obese is more likely to develop osteoarthritis of the knee (between 2.5 times and 4.6 times according to their BMI (body mass index)).[2, 3, 4]

You can calculate your BMI to find out if you are classed as overweight or obese by going online to www.nhs.uk/live-well/healthy-weight/bmi-calculator. This website can tell you if you are overweight, a healthy weight or underweight.

For those who are just 3 kg (6 or 7 lb) above their BMI, it's surprising how much difference it can make to your mobility to lose that amount. Many of us have fluctuating weight and if you become aware of when knees or hips start niggling again, it might be time to lose a few pounds again. If you've already lost weight you may know how to do this quite easily by cutting down, eating salads, and soups (in winter), to lower the calorie count.

The force through the knees

Dr Tom Margham, GP, explains, 'Every time we take a step, the force of three to six times our bodyweight goes through our knees, so the link between weight and load through the knee is clear. If you are overweight, reducing your body mass index (BMI) by two units reduces the risk of developing osteoarthritis in the knee by 50 per cent. For a woman of average height this equates to approximately 5 kg (12 lb) weight loss, which is a modest target.'

He claims, 'Losing around 5 per cent of body weight or at least 6 kg (almost 1 stone/14 lb) leads to noticeable improvement in the way people move and feel but may not obviously reduce pain. Research shows that combinations of diet and exercise lead to:

- more weight loss
- less pain
- better function
- faster walking speed
- longer walking distance and
- better health-related quality of life
  than diet and exercise alone.'

Even a small amount of weight loss will give relief to your knees. Research has shown that losing as little as 5 kg (11 lb) can improve joint health and cut the risk of osteoarthritis of the knee by 50 per cent in women.[5] For every pound of weight lost, there is a four-pound reduction in the load exerted on the knee for each step that occurs during daily activities,[6] and vice-versa for every extra pound you gain.

An article in *Healthbeat*, a Harvard Medical publication,[7] claimed:

'When you walk across level ground, the force on your knees is the equivalent of 1½ times your body weight. That means a 200-pound* man will put 300 pounds** of pressure on his knees with each step.'

*200 lb = 90.7 kg, 14 stone+ **300 lb = 136 kg, 21 stone+.

Stairs and hills

Add an incline, and the pressure is even greater. The force on each knee is two to three times your body weight when you go up and down stairs, and four to five times your body weight when you squat to tie a shoelace or pick up an item you have dropped.

Losing a few pounds can go a long way towards reducing the pressure on your knees – and protecting them. For example, research has proven that a sustained 4.5–6.8 kg (10 to 15 lb or 1 stone 1 lb) weight loss in obese young people can translate to a much lower risk of osteoarthritis later in life.[7] And as always, prevention is better than cure.

Dr Tom Margham, GP, suggests that just losing 5 kg (11 lb) can bring an improvement in symptoms. 'Joints are living tissue which repair themselves, but they become overwhelmed by stresses and strain, which result in pain. This can be due to biomechanics – the force moving through a joint in an unusual way, overuse of the joint through activity, or being overweight.'

Chapter 3

Finding exercise to suit you

The benefits of exercise cannot be exaggerated. It doesn't matter what you do as long as you do some activity that is suitable for you. Most people can improve their muscle strength, whatever level they start from. The days of resting when you have pain or discomfort are over: inactivity is recognised as causing more problems than it solves.

Start gradually and build it up, however little it is. If you feel reluctant and are worried about pain, be assured that exercise can make you feel really good.

Health experts claim that we should exercise on at least five days a week for around 30 minutes. Depending on your ability, it is good to do enough exercise to get out of breath. If exercise is difficult it can be broken down into 10-minute slots (three times a day). Activity counts as exercise, so doing a bit of gardening, going for a gentle walk, or anything that gets you moving, is just as valid as playing a sport or attending a yoga class.

The benefits of exercise

- Exercise builds up and strengthens muscles which support and protect the joints.
- It improves circulation, taking more blood around the body and to the extremities (fingers and toes), and keeps you

warm. Professor Sir Sam Everington explains, 'When the weather is cold, the periphery shut down so that our hands and feet get cold first. This is nature's way of preserving the core of our body, so the way to counteract this process is by activity, which is like turning on our own central heating system.'

- Burning up calories through exercise is a great way to lose weight.
- Activity is good for the heart and strengthens the cardiovascular system.
- Keeping active and moving a lot maintains and improves mobility.
- Exercises designed for people with osteoarthritis improve balance and help to prevent falls.
- Weight-bearing exercise maintains bone density, lessening the chances of getting osteoporosis (where the bones become porous, full of holes and very brittle).
- Activity and exercises make people feel good as they increase blood flow to the brain, and release *endorphins* in the body, the so-called happy hormones that can ease anxiety and mild depression.[1]
- Exercise in groups is a social activity which can improve our mood by enabling us to get out of the house and meet people.

Why exercise is good for osteoarthritis

Dr Roger Wolman explains, 'Natural balance awareness is lost because the sensors don't work efficiently inside a joint that has deteriorated. By building up muscle strength you improve the function of the joint and retrain it in balance awareness.

'Exercise also slows down the deterioration in joints that occurs due to ageing. If a joint is painful, we tend to do less exercise, increasing the pace of deterioration, so if you can't jog try something else such as cycling or rowing exercises. Exercises in water, such as walking, take the stress out of the joint.' (See the section on hydrotherapy later in this chapter, page 36.)

Exercise that's right for you

It doesn't have to be expensive and you don't have to go somewhere to do it. Sometimes you can add a walk into your day rather than taking the car or getting the bus. And don't be put off if you are less mobile – everyone can find some exercise that is suitable for them at every level. There are plenty of exercises that can be modified to your limits, including chair yoga for those who cannot easily stand (see details on page 41).

It is important to manage osteoarthritis, rather than ignore it. This doesn't mean giving up the hobbies and activities you love but doing them sensibly. It's tempting to avoid doing any activity due to fear of aggravating painful and swollen joints. Doing nothing could make them much worse.

Start slowly and be sensible

Dr Tom Margham, GP, and former Arthritis Research UK's primary care lead, emphasises that it's important to be sensible and build up exercise gradually. 'It's always important to prepare with warm-up exercises, rather than launching into vigorous activity. It's quite common to respond to any pain by stopping immediately. It's important to differentiate between pain that is due to injury and the natural discomfort that results after exercise when you're not used to it.'

However, a word of warning from Sammy Margo, Chartered Physiotherapist, who says, 'Individuals should find the right level of activity for them so that they don't do too much or too little. Some people could do six 5-minute walks a day, as opposed to a 30-minute chunk of exercise which could be excessive for them.'

Some people get osteoarthritis from doing too much sport or fitness activity, so a happy medium is preferable. It is important to stay mobile and keep up exercise of some kind to both prevent osteoarthritis and stop it getting any worse.

Sensible precautions

If you play tennis or other active sports, wear good shoes with a lot of support, and sports supports for your arthritic joints – wraps and/or braces for knees, especially, and wrists which are available online, at sports shops and in some large chemists. If you have, for example, osteoarthritis in the knee, it wouldn't be sensible to play long games of tennis five times a week. Find the level that suits you as continuing exercise is good for you.

What sort of exercise is helpful?

Dr Tom Margham, recommends a mixture of:

- **Resistance** – for strength and joint stability. Any exercise that works to strengthen muscles. This can mean working against a weight or resistance band, or the biggest source of free resistance – gravity! For example, moving from sitting to standing or partial squats are resistance exercises.
- **Aerobic exercise** – for fitness endurance and mood. Just walking for half an hour a day builds up stamina and helps the heart. Being out of breath is not a problem as it indicates that you are putting effort in. It increases the body's demand for oxygen, strengthens the heart, lungs and circulation by preventing blood clotting, lowering blood pressure and raising the level of protective cholesterol. Aerobic exercise includes walking, running, dancing, swimming, tennis and spinning.
- **Flexibility** – for balance, range of movement and co-ordination. Tai chi and qigong (chi kung) include some of

the best exercises for improving balance. Some movements in qigong and tai chi involve standing on one leg (see Chapter 4).

Activities to consider

- **Cycling** is good for strengthening muscles in the thighs (particularly the hamstrings). However, it's important not to overdo this and cause strain. Cycling doesn't have to mean getting on a bike and battling the traffic and weather. It's just as good to cycle on an exercise bike in the safety of your own home – it means you are more likely to get round to doing it and experience the benefits to the muscles and the knees. It's no good saying that you enjoy cycling and going out about six times a year.
- **Swimming** is gentle exercise which helps the lower part of the body to relax and builds up muscle. Rheumatologist, Dr Rod Hughes, comments, 'Swimming is excellent for arthritis in the lower limbs (hips, knees and feet) – but not so much for upper limbs as it can put strain on the neck or arms.' (See also the section on hydrotherapy on page 36.)
- **Dancing**, particularly any type which involves the arms and hands, such as Indian style. Ballroom dancing is enjoying renewed popularity because of *Strictly Come Dancing*, so if you enjoy it, do as much as you can but be careful of wearing very high heels for long, as they can make your aches and pains much worse.
- **Walking**. Walking is good for your heart, lungs, and joints, so take every opportunity you can, such as taking the stairs instead of the lift or walking to the station. If you try to avoid stairs because of your knees, think about adding in a walk instead of going by car or public transport. Just 20 minutes walking five times a week is good for your heart, helps you lose weight and keeps you mobile.

- **Yoga** is particularly good for stretching and flexing muscles and making your body stronger.
- **Tai chi and chi kung (qigong)** are often practised by older people and there are classes around the country where the maximum age is within the 90s. It encourages gentle movement and balance.
- **Pilates** is very popular these days and there are often classes designed especially for the over-60s. It helps to improve your core muscles and takes the strain off your back – see Chapter 4, page 42.

Other activities – not strictly exercise

- **Knitting or sewing** is excellent for keeping your hands moving and flexible.
- **Gardening** can keep people occupied, happy and active, but it's important to bend correctly from the knees and not cause strain on your back. Trying to be mindful while gardening means that you work within your limits. If it hurts to dig or to do the weeding, it's important to stop.
- **Piano playing** is excellent for fingers because of the exercise it gives them. So, if you've got an opportunity and you know how to play a bit, it's worth getting back to it. Or taking it up for the first time.

Wake up your body every day!

Whole body tapping is a great way to wake up your body in the morning and get the circulation going. You can tap with your fingertips from top to toe, starting with the top of your head, your neck and shoulders, down both arms, on your front and where you can reach on your back, down both legs and onto your feet. It makes you feel good and more able to start some exercise. You can find videos of body tapping on YouTube.

Exercises to do anywhere, any time

There are plenty of exercises you can do in your own time at home or anywhere which are designed to help people with osteoarthritis, and a selection are listed here.

Spiky massage balls

These balls are cheap and easy to find on the internet and can be used to massage hands, feet and backs. The 9-cm size is adequate, and you can squeeze the balls in the hands, roll your feet back and forth on them for a deep foot massage, or use them under your back. If you've got a particular area of your back that is bothering you, lie down on the floor or a suitable massage table and move around on top of the ball for a deep massage. They get the circulation going, relieve muscle tension and help to ease aches and pains.

Exercises for knees

Step ups

Step onto the bottom step of stairs with your right foot. Bring up your left foot, step down with your right foot, followed by your left foot. Repeat with each leg until you get short of breath. Hold on to the banister if necessary. As you improve, try to increase the number of steps you can achieve in one minute and the height of the step.

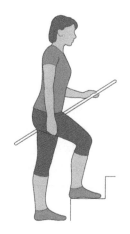

Sit/stands

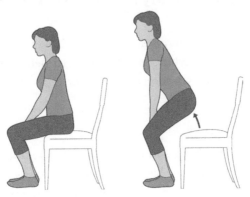

Sit on a chair. Without using your hands for support, stand up and then sit back down. Make sure each movement is slow and controlled. Repeat for one minute. As you improve, try to increase the number of sit/stands you can do in one minute and try the exercise from lower chairs or the bottom two steps of a staircase.

Knee to chest

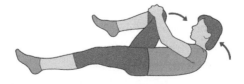

Lie on the floor or other firm surface (the bed might be too soft) with your legs out straight and your hands by the side of your body. Bend one knee and put your hands around it as shown, pulling it gently towards you as much as you can. Lift your head and see how close you can get it to the bent knee.

Straight-leg raise (sitting)

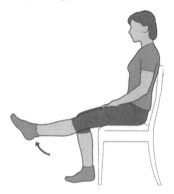

Sit well back in a chair, with good posture. Straighten and raise one leg. Hold for a slow count to 10, then slowly lower your leg. If you can do this easily, try it with light weights on your ankles and with your toes pointing towards you.

Try doing this while relaxing and watching TV.

Straight leg raise (lying)

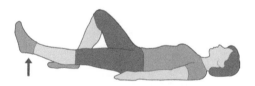

Bend one leg at the knee, as shown. Hold the other leg straight and lift the related foot just off the surface you are lying on. Hold for a slow count of 5, then lower. Repeat five times with each leg.

Try doing it in the morning and at night while lying in bed.

Knee leg stretch

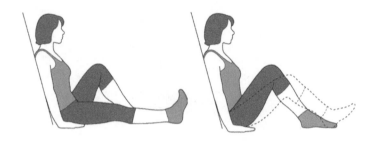

Sit on the floor with your legs stretched out in front.
(a) Keeping your foot to the floor, slowly bend one knee until you feel it being comfortably stretched. Hold for five seconds.
(b) Straighten your leg as far as you can and hold for five seconds.

Repeat 10 times with each leg.

Knee leg cross

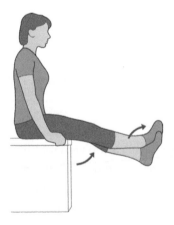

Sit on the edge of a table, bed or other surface. Cross your ankles over. Push your front leg backwards and back leg forwards against each other until the thigh muscles become tense. Hold for 10 seconds, then relax. Switch legs and repeat. Do four sets with each leg.

Knee squats

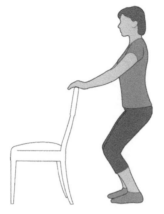

Hold onto a chair or work surface for support. Squat down until your kneecaps cover your big toes. Return to standing.

Start with one or two of these and try to increase up to 10 times. As you improve, try to squat a little further. Don't bend your knees beyond a right angle.

Exercises for hips

Hip flexion (strengthening)

Hold onto a work surface and march slowly on the spot to bring your knees up towards your chest alternately. Don't bring your thigh above 90 degrees.

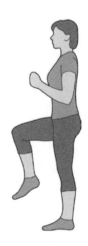

Heel to buttock exercise (strengthening)

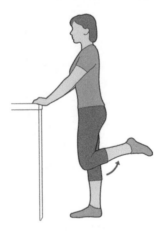

Bend one knee and pull your heel up towards your bottom. Keep your knees in line and the kneecap of the bent leg pointing towards the floor. Hold on to something solid if you have problems with balancing.

Hip extension (strengthening)

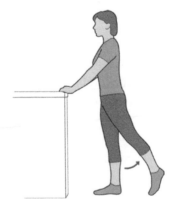

Move one leg backwards, keeping your knee straight. Clench the buttock on that side tightly and hold for five seconds. Don't lean forwards. Hold onto a chair or work surface for support.

Hip abduction (strengthening)

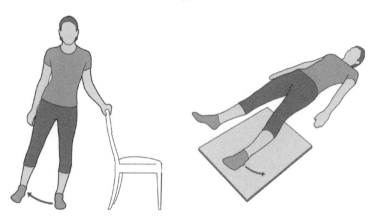

(a) Lift one leg sideways, being careful not to rotate it outwards. Hold for five seconds and bring it back slowly, keeping your body straight throughout. Hold onto a chair or work surface for support. (b) Alternatively, do this while lying down.

Mini squat (strengthening)

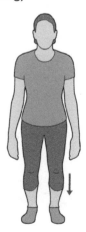

Squat down gradually until your knees are above your toes. Hold for a count of 5 if possible. Hold on to a work surface for support if you need to.

Hips external rotation

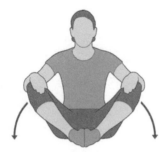

Sit on the floor, bend your knees and put the soles of your feet together. Gently push your upper legs outwards towards the floor.

Short arc quadriceps exercise (strengthening)

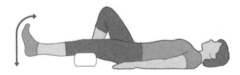

Lie down, with one leg bent for support as shown, and place a rolled-up towel under the other knee. Keep the back of your thigh on the towel and straighten your knee to raise your foot off the floor. Hold for five seconds and then lower slowly.

Quadriceps exercise (strengthening)

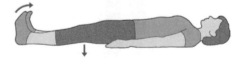

Lie down flat on your back (or if you prefer you can do this while sitting). Pull your toes and ankles towards you, while keeping your legs straight and pushing your knees firmly against the floor. You should feel the tightness in the front of your legs. Hold for five seconds and relax.

Stomach exercise (strengthening/stabilising)

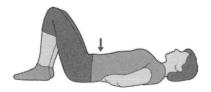

Lie on your back with your knees bent. Put your hands under the small of your back and pull your belly button down towards the floor. Hold for a count of 20.

Hips external rotation (stretch)

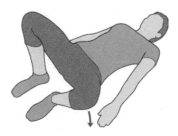

Lie down, bend your knees and put your feet flat on the floor. Press your knees down towards the floor using your hands as needed. Alternatively, lie on your back and part your knees, keeping your feet together.

Take the movement up to the point you feel a stretch, hold for around 10 seconds and relax. Repeat up to 10 times.

Exercises for hands

Many people have osteoarthritis in the thumb joints and fingers. These exercises help to improve flexibility and mobility in the fingers and thumbs and are suitable for everyone to do.

Splayed hands

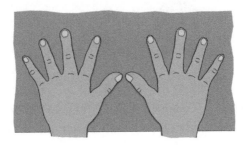

Spread your hands out so that the fingers are splayed and place them on a flat surface, such as a table or desk.

Strengthening and flexing

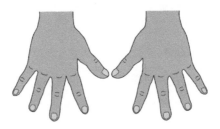

Stretch out your fingers in a similar way without putting them on a surface. You can do this in bed, or anytime during the day to strengthen the muscles in your hands. Try to be aware of when you are clenching your fists at any time and relax your hands.

Squeeze ball

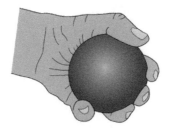

Get hold of a soft ball made of foam or a stress ball (the size of a tennis ball) and squeeze it regularly with each hand. Preferably support your arm while doing this so that you don't put pressure on your arms. It helps to improve your grip and the strength of your hand muscles as well as the mobility in fingers.

You can do this several times a day.

Thumb to fingers

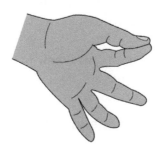

Turn your hand palm upwards and move your thumb over to touch your little finger; take it back and then move to the other three fingers in turn. This may be painful for an arthritic thumb joint at first, but it helps to strengthen the joint and improve mobility.

Making a fist

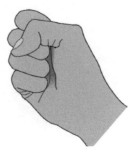

Make a fist of one hand and open again. Repeat up to 10 times and then do the same with the other hand.

More ideas for exercising hands

- Play the piano – or pretend to play 'air' piano, exercising your fingers.
- Knitting is great exercise.
- Shake your hands vigorously as often as you can to release tension. This may hurt at first but try to persist.

See Chapter 9 for other ideas about how to use computers and take the strain off your hands and body in general.

Gentle exercises for the less mobile

We tend to live much more sedentary lifestyles these days, and it takes effort and discipline to go out and exercise. Some people take up exercise as they get older in a bid to beat old age and immobility, while others may think 'I'm past it now, I can't start exercising at my age'.

If you have problems with mobility there are still plenty of exercises that you can use – such as chair yoga, or other exercises that you can do within your own limits. So, start with gentle exercise that suits you.

Professor Sir Sam Everington asserts: 'Inactivity causes 10 years loss of life. An 80-year-old who is in bed for 10 days loses 10 per cent of their muscle strength, which is equivalent to being inactive for 10 years.'

Anyone with good muscle strength and bone mass will fare better when they are confined to bed for a while than those who have poor muscle strength and bone mass.

Chair exercises

For those people who find standing very difficult, there are plenty of exercises that can be done while sitting in a chair. It's possible to give the body a mini workout from this position.

- While seated lift the lower half of each leg in turn and bend it upwards. Flex the foot, pointing the toe and then flattening the foot in the air.
- Put your feet flat on the floor and lift the heels first and then the toes, giving them a workout.
- Hunch your shoulders up to your ears and back down again. This can be done in a circular motion, first forwards and then backwards.
- Look slowly from left to right, trying to look a bit further behind you each time, making sure your shoulders are relaxed.

Also read about chair yoga in Chapter 4 (page 41), as it is a great alternative for the less mobile.

Exercises to improve balance

Hold on to a firm piece of furniture that won't move, such as the kitchen sink. Make sure there are no knives or other dangerous objects nearby. Raise each foot off the floor one by one – lift the left foot, followed by the right foot. Then do this with one hand off the furniture and progress to taking both hands off when you feel confident.

Exercise in water – hydrotherapy

Hydrotherapy has become a component part of medical treatment for arthritis in the UK, and pools are accessible, for at least limited periods, to both NHS and private patients in hospitals, and also at some health clubs. Access to hydrotherapy for NHS patients depends on the local CCG (Community Care Group) facilities.

'It's important to do exercise while in the hydrotherapy pool,' Dr Rod Hughes explains. 'The warm water soothes muscles and enables people to do exercises they couldn't do on dry land, such as squats and lifting legs.'

Being in warm water makes it easier to fully stretch and strengthen the muscles. The warmth relieves pain and provides enjoyable relaxation. The water should be very warm so that it feels like a bath. For people who are quite active, there are often local aqua classes which are inexpensive, although it's worth checking out how warm the pool is.

Chapter 4

Exercises to protect and strengthen your body

Dr Tom Margham, GP in Tower Hamlets and former Arthritis Research UK's primary care lead, considers both yoga and tai chi to be excellent for people as they get older, whether or not they have arthritis:

'There are a lot of movements from side to side in tai chi and yoga. People don't habitually take steps from side to side, so they lose this skill due to sitting in one place all the time. It means they can't cope with being off balance and are more prone to falling.

'Also one of the first things to go when we get older is rotation of the joints. It also becomes difficult to put the leg out to the side and extend the joint. Many older people also have weak muscles in their bottoms.'

The 'glutes' (gluteus maximus, medius and minimus muscles) located in the side of the buttocks are the biggest muscles in the body, connected to the tailbone (coccyx) and surrounding bones. They have many roles:

- keeping the trunk of the body upright
- helping us to walk upstairs
- responsibility for the movement of the hip and the thigh.

Breathing

We need to remember that breath is the life force, providing our bodies with energy. It influences the nervous system and the brain. Yet we breathe in and out without giving it a second thought, but how deeply? Shallow breathing is responsible for many health issues and yet is completely normal for so many people, especially when they are tense.

Deep breathing is a vital aspect of tai chi, yoga and Alexander Technique and is calming, energising and health-giving. It increases the flow of blood round the body and helps our bodies to relax.

Tai chi and qigong

There couldn't be a more suitable form of exercise for people as they get older. Millions of Chinese people have been practising tai chi (and qigong) for centuries and they believe that it rejuvenates them and leads to a prolonged life. And now it is gaining popularity in the UK, especially with older people for whom the benefits are becoming more and more recognised.

Tai chi has always been associated with keeping healthy, energising and repairing the body. The exercises are not strenuous but gentle and so are well suited to older people and those with osteoarthritis.

Benefits of tai chi and qigong

- Relaxes and calms the mind, improves concentration and brings greater body awareness.
- Improves and maintains suppleness and mobility.
- Gently tones muscles.
- Improves balance and posture, which both deteriorate with age.
- Maintains stability and flexibility in the joints.
- Boosts circulation throughout the body.

The slow gentle movements stimulate the body's energy or

chi and massage the meridians – the lines which run through the body in the acupuncture system, and give a complete inner and outer workout.

Tai chi involves learning and following a particular sequence of movements, rather like learning a flowing dance. Focusing on these movements and remembering them helps with concentration and allows the mind to cut off from everyday concerns.

While similar, qigong (or chi kung/gung) was originally developed to improve health. It consists of a series of repetitive gentle movements which are easy to learn and follow so it's possible to do them with eyes closed for a really relaxing experience.

Research endorsements

There has been a good deal of research into the effectiveness of tai chi in preventing falls in elderly people.[1, 2, 3, 4]

A US study at Tufts University in Boston compared the health benefits of tai chi with those of physical therapy,[5] in 204 people of around 60 years old who had symptomatic and radiographic knee arthritis. After 12 weeks the tai chi group saw a greater improvement in pain and functioning than the physical therapy group, as well as experiencing improved mental health and lower rates of depression. In addition, a review of 66 (randomised controlled) trials of both tai chi and qigong showed many health benefits, including better bone health and improved prevention of falls.[6]

Suitable for everyone

Check out classes before you attend – tai chi was originally a martial art but is now frequently practised in a non-aggressive and gentle therapeutic manner, which is more suitable for people with osteoarthritis.

There is no competitive element so people can go at their own pace and to their own level. If they have difficulty standing for long periods they can hold on to a table or chair or can do some of the exercises sitting down.

There are tai chi and qigong classes all over the UK, and there are occasionally practice trials on the NHS. Generally, there is a small fee to pay, which is not excessive. To find classes, look for advertisements on library noticeboards and local newsagents' shop windows, in health food stores, or online. Find out more in Further information at the end of the book (page 134).

Yoga

Photographs in magazines may give the impression that yoga is only for the young, but this doesn't reflect the benefits it has for everyone. Yoga is not competitive, and you do what you can at your level.

Participants are encouraged to be aware of how their body feels and adapt their movements accordingly.

These benefits include:

- exercising every muscle in the body
- improving balance
- firming up and strengthening muscles
- keeping the body supple and flexible
- helping you to relax and reduce stress levels.

It's vital to find a class that is appropriate for you with an instructor who is empathetic to your needs, and sometimes there are classes run specifically for the over 60s. There are many different types of yoga, but the British Wheel of Yoga recommends Hatha Yoga as a safe and therapeutic form that is still challenging enough to provide all the benefits. Yoga suits people of all ages and sizes, and if you're not supple it's an even better reason to do it.

Chair yoga

For people who find getting down on the floor too difficult and have problems with standing for too long, chair yoga is an excellent way to feel the advantages. Participants either sit on a chair or use it for support and can adapt postures to suit their ability.

Richard Kravetz, a British Wheel of Yoga instructor and a well-respected teacher of chair yoga, explains, 'Chair yoga helps people to stay safe from injury while improving mobility, flexibility and strength. The chair helps people to compensate for lack of balance and strength and empowers them to be more confident in movement. It enables people to gain the really positive aspects of yoga, which can enrich lives and enable people to find direction in life.'

Relaxation and breathing

Not only does yoga bring physical benefits which stretch and tone the body but breathing and relaxation also play a major part in sessions. People are encouraged to focus on their breathing because it is very common to breathe too shallowly.

Deep breathing with an emphasis on taking air into the diaphragm increases the intake of oxygen, improving the flow of energy and the circulation of blood and lymph throughout the body. This helps to relieve tightness in the chest and in the muscles and is relaxing and calming.

The roots of yoga go back thousands of years in Indian culture and it is integral to the Ayurvedic system of medicine which has a holistic approach rather than a purely medical one. The word yoga means union as its aim is to unite mind, body and spirit for health and wellbeing.

Richard Kravetz warns not to do anything that causes pain. 'Use props such as blocks, bolsters, cushions or blankets for extra support to minimise discomfort. There are plenty of pain-free ways of practising a range of movements and lubricating the joints through the exercise.

'There is a lot you can do for arthritic fingers, such as opening and closing hands, separating fingers and also massaging them,' he continues. 'I encourage people to listen to their body and adapt or soften movements to avoid pain or inflammation. Many health problems can improve by doing yoga.'

Pilates

Pilates took the UK by storm in the late 1990s to early 2000s and now there are classes everywhere. Joseph Pilates developed it almost 100 years ago to help him to fight the ill health which had dogged him since childhood. He ended up living until 87 and then died as a result of a fire in his New York studio.

It's important to check out classes for Pilates, because some are quite challenging but there are plenty of sessions for people over 60 and some specifically for those with osteoarthritis.

Pilates consists of small precise movements practised lying down or standing, which help you to become aware of the core muscles supporting the spine.

The benefits of Pilates are that it:

- helps to improve posture and flexibility
- lengthens and tones muscle
- strengthens joints
- reduces stress
- eases pain.

Teacher, author and video presenter of Pilates, Lynne Robinson, explains, 'Pilates is the perfect choice of exercise for anyone with arthritis. It teaches you to be aware of the alignment of all your joints before you start an exercise and while you perform it. Your movements are slow and controlled so there's no strain on the joints. The focus is to mobilise the joints and strengthen the muscles surrounding them so that they are supported.

'The combination of correct alignment, balanced muscles and good stability means there's less wear and tear on joints. The gentle movements encourage the production of synovial fluid to lubricate the joints. Pilates can be mat based or in the studio. In both, your teacher will ensure you are in supported positions while you exercise, enabling you to enjoy the movements.'

Brigitte Tetlow, Pilates teacher, explains, 'Keeping mobile when you have osteoarthritis is extremely important. Exercise lubricates joints, maintains cartilage, and strengthens muscles. It improves your overall health, fitness and wellbeing.

'Pilates can help to reduce pain in the joints, increase your range of movement and flexibility and improve your strength. When you have osteoarthritis, the cartilage breaks down so that bone is no longer protected. Bone rubs on bone causing pain. By mobilising the joints, you increase the synovial fluid which lubricates the joints and makes everything work better.

'It's always important to inform your teacher of any limitations you have and modify exercises accordingly. You should work at your own level depending on your flexibility and any pain you have.

'It's good to have a positive approach to exercise and the benefits it can bring. Imagine an old car rusting in the garage. Give it some oil and petrol and get it moving again and it will run well. The same applies to us.'

The Alexander technique

The Alexander technique is all about awareness of how you are using your body and putting unnecessary strain on it, which can be described as mindfulness in activity. The Alexander technique teacher aims to encourage this awareness and leave you with the tools to prevent unnecessary physical stress and tension.

Our bodies were not designed to sit at computers, slouch on the sofa or drive a car for long journeys. You need to stand up and move around regularly, or even do some exercises to loosen up your body.

The Alexander technique makes you aware of how you are using your body when sitting, standing, walking and lying down. It is all about becoming mindful when active, being aware of *how* you are moving, sitting, standing etc, and whether or not it is putting strain on your body. By reducing strain, you can avoid aggravating vulnerable areas or making the muscles and joints ache.

One relaxing tip is to try the semi-supine position, often used in the Alexander technique (see below). Lie on a carpeted floor or a massage table, but not on a bed because you will sink into it. Put a couple of paperback books under your head but adjust these to suit – you may need thinner books, or you may want to add one. Your knees should be bent but not touching each other and your feet should be flat on the surface. Stay there for up to 20 minutes with your hands beside you, a few inches away from your body or resting on your stomach. Think about where it is that you are holding tension, working from your head downwards while gradually relaxing.

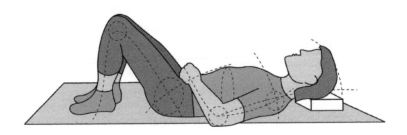

The semi-supine position

Ian O'Donnell, Alexander Technique teacher, comments, 'We often put more effort than is physically required into our daily activities. A prime example is when we brush our teeth.

'Think about how tightly you are gripping the toothbrush, or if you're scrunching up your shoulders and generally tensing up when there is no need. Are you hunching your shoulders or holding the phone with your neck? When using a computer, are your feet flat on the floor and is your back comfortably supported?'

Be aware of the following activities and consider whether you can make a change that eases the strain or pain:

- carrying shopping
- doing housework, especially using the vacuum cleaner
- getting in and out of the car
- driving
- sitting at the computer, mobile phone or laptop (see Chapter 9)
- playing sport
- going up and down stairs
- gardening
- walking along the road.

Ian O'Donnell explains, 'Believe it or not, when your head protrudes forward it increases the strain on your neck, shoulders and back. The aim is to get your head nicely balanced on top of your spine and decrease the load that your neck and shoulders have to contend with. This allows your neck to be released and the pain and tension in your shoulders to be reduced.'

Chapter 5

What is healthy eating?

New diets make media headlines all the time, but the simple principle is that if we don't burn up the calories we take in, most people put on weight. Exercise and activity are the answer to keeping us fit and healthy to fight disease as well as controlling weight. There are loads of faddy diets and plenty of controversy about the best way to lose weight, but the following guidelines are recommended as a useful starting point:

- Reduce portion sizes and cut down on calories.
- Exchange sugary snacks and drinks, pastries and biscuits for healthy snacks like nuts, fruit and sugar-free yoghurts.
- Include vegetables, a moderate amount of fruit, wholegrains such as brown rice, wholemeal bread and pasta, pulses (lentils, beans and split peas), chicken, turkey and fish in your daily diet.

Making a lifestyle change and eating more of the above on a long-term basis works better than following a diet for a while and then going back to eating as you did before.

A well-known diet is the 5:2 approach, where you fast for two days a week and eat normally for five. Many people are put off this diet because of the fasting. However, a variation of this idea can be effective – if you have two light days with fewer calories and five days where you eat normal (healthy) meals, it is very likely that you will eat less overall, and experience gradual loss of weight.

As mentioned in Chapter 2, it is more helpful to tackle weight loss in increments so that when you have lost say, 3.18 kg or half a stone, it can spur you on to losing the next 3 kg or half a stone and so on. This takes time and results shouldn't be expected in a few weeks because that means putting undue pressure on yourself which can end in giving up altogether.

Some people seem more motivated to lose weight when they attend a slimming club (such as Weight Watchers or Slimming World) which can produce very good results.

Is the Mediterranean diet good for arthritis?

One diet that is claimed to be particularly good for health is the Mediterranean diet. It is forecast that by 2040 (if current trends continue) Spain will have the highest life expectancy in the world at 87.4 years, taking over from Japan which topped the table in 2016.[1] This is said to be due to the Mediterranean diet eaten in Spain.

The good news is that this diet is particularly good for those with osteoarthritis. Researchers at the University of Kent looked into the effects of the Mediterranean diet on people with osteoarthritis for the UK charity, Arthritis Action. They found that inflammation of the joints and cartilage decay decreased in those participants who ate the healthy diet.[2] They also gained greater knee and hip mobility and on average lost 2.2 per cent in weight.

So what is the Mediterranean diet and why is it so healthy? It is a plant-based diet, consisting of plenty of fruit and vegetables, pulses, beans, olive oil, nuts and fish. It may also consist of chicken and turkey (white meats) but is low in red meat (see the Pyramid on page 48). Not only is it healthy but it also tastes great. Fruit and vegetables are good for you generally, but they have been found to be particularly helpful in easing knee pain in older people.[3]

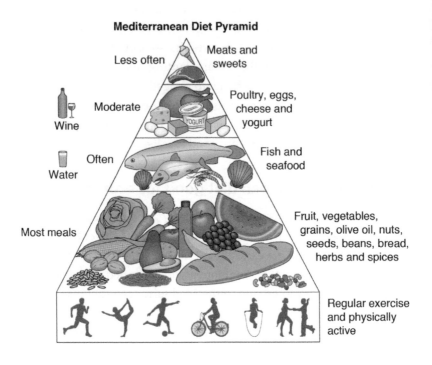

Mediterranean Diet Pyramid

Less often — Meats and sweets

Wine

Moderate — Poultry, eggs, cheese and yogurt

Water

Often — Fish and seafood

Most meals — Fruit, vegetables, grains, olive oil, nuts, seeds, beans, bread, herbs and spices

Regular exercise and physically active

The Mediterranean diet typically consists of:

- **Healthy fats**: The Mediterranean diet is packed full of healthy fats – unsaturated fats, which are in olive oil and oily fish (salmon, herring, mackerel, tuna). In the UK we have a tendency to eat a lot of saturated fats. The NHS website advises that an average man of 19 to 64 years old should only eat 30 g of saturated fats a day. Typically these fats are in butter, ghee, suet, lard, palm oil, cakes and biscuits, fatty meats, sausages, bacon and cured meats (salami, pancetta, chorizo), cheeses, pastries and pies, cream, ice cream and chocolate.

- **Less sugar**: The Mediterranean diet is less packed with sugar than many British foods. Quite apart from cakes, biscuits, chocolate and desserts containing added sugar, there are plenty of hidden sugars in processed and canned foods.
- **Nutritious**: It's a diet high in vitamins and antioxidants which also have a positive effect on those with osteoarthritis.
- **Olive oil**: One of the best aspects of the Mediterranean diet is the consumption of olive oil, which is high in antioxidants and is claimed to have an anti-inflammatory effect on the body, due to the oleic acid, a mono-saturated fat. Healthy tip: eat uncooked cold-pressed extra virgin oil by drizzling it on your salad or vegetables.

Understand healthy eating

One of the best ways of maintaining weight loss is to become more knowledgeable about nutrition and what constitutes healthy eating, and this can be better understood by knowing more about the food groups. Rather than following short-term diets, if you change the way you eat on a long-term basis you can lose pounds gradually and maintain weight loss.

The three main food groups are:

- carbohydrates
- proteins
- fats.

It is important to eat food from all of these groups, and not focus just on one. Low-carb diets may prove effective but are controversial because health experts believe that the body needs each of the main food groups.

Carbohydrates

The main fuel for the body, carbohydrates are required for energy, but these days most people eat far too many fast-releasing carbohydrates rather than slow-release ones.

The following are all carbohydrates: rice, pasta, pizza base, potatoes, bread, oats, noodles, couscous, cereals, vegetables, fresh fruit, wholegrains, sugar, honey.

- Slow-releasing or complex carbohydrates provide energy over a longer period than fast-releasing carbs. These include wholegrains such as brown rice, brown bread, wholewheat pasta, vegetables and fresh fruit. All of these foods are high in fibre, which is good for healthy digestion.
- Fast-releasing carbohydrates give a quick burst of energy followed by a slump that many people will be familiar with. These include sugar, white flour, white rice, potatoes, sweets, biscuits, cakes, chocolate, and some sugary fruits – bananas, dates, raisins and dried fruits.

Proteins

Protein is essential for growth and repair of the body and maintains good health, so it is essential in the diet. GP Dr Tom Margham, also former Arthritis Research UK's primary care lead, claims, 'Many older people enjoy a diet of tea and toast, which means they are not eating enough protein. Consequently, they lose muscle mass and as osteoarthritis also results in muscle loss, they are more likely to have pain and/or fall over.'

Good quality protein is found in eggs, fish, cheese, chicken, lean beef and lamb, soya beans, beans and legumes (chickpeas, lentils), broccoli, spinach, corn, yoghurt, brown rice, quinoa and pumpkin and sunflower seeds.

Fats

There is plenty of confusion about fats because there are different types and they are sometimes not fully understood. Not all fats are bad for us, but some are.

Polyunsaturated or essential fats

Essential fatty acids (long chain polyunsaturated oils or LCPs for short), are required for healthy brain development and function, and keep the joints well oiled, which is important for osteoarthritis. The two main types are omega-3 and omega-6.

Omega-3s are found in:

- oily fish – such as mackerel, salmon, tuna, sardines, herrings
- flaxseed oil or linseeds
- hemp seed / oil
- pumpkin seeds
- walnuts.

Omega-6s are found in:

- sunflower seeds / oil
- sesame seeds / oil
- corn oil
- soy beans.

In our British diet we get too many omega-6s and not enough omega-3s. This is largely because we aren't natural lovers of oily fish like the Scandinavians. And there are also problems with mercury and plastics getting into fish, which put off a lot of people from eating them.

Important tip:

The amount of omega-6s to -3s we should be eating is 4:1 but in recent years the ratio for the amount we consume has gone up to 16:1 or even higher. Registered Medical Herbalist, Chris Etheridge, explains, 'Many nut oils are high in omega-6 fatty acids that are pro-inflammatory, compared with omega-3 which is anti-inflammatory. We currently have diets too high in omega-6 compared with omega-3, so it is suggested that reducing omega-6 and increasing omega-3 intake will be beneficial for controlling inflammatory processes.'[4]

Monounsaturated fats

The foods that contain mono-unsaturated fats are generally considered to be healthy – avocado, olive oil, and some nuts (e.g. cashews, walnuts) and seeds.

Saturated fats

Most people are aware that butter, hard cheese, cream, full cream milk, and fatty meat products contain fats that should not be eaten in large quantities. The NHS claims on its website that people in the UK eat too many saturated fats which are believed to increase LDL, the type of   cholesterol which can lead to increased likelihood of strokes and heart disease. It recommends that men should not have more than 30 g of saturated fat a day, women 20 g, and children less.

Hydrogenated fats (or trans fats)

These have been phased out in many foods now but it's still worth reading the labels. They increase cholesterol levels, clog arteries and lead to heart disease and strokes. They have no nutritional use in the body and block its ability to take up polyunsaturated oils (see above). They are typically in processed foods such as pies, gravy mixes, biscuits, cakes, margarine and other spreads, ice cream, pre-packaged foods, and fast food such as burgers.

Enjoying a tipple

It's no secret that a lot of older people have been drinking too much alcohol for years and consider it a normal part of their lives. Figures published in May 2017[5] showed that more than half a million adults aged between 55 and 74 were admitted to English hospitals with alcohol-related injuries, diseases or conditions, an increase of 64 per cent in a decade.

Drinking guidelines were reduced for men a few years ago and the recommended maximum is now the same as for women – 14 units per week. A unit is one small glass of wine, one measure of spirits or half a pint of beer and is equivalent to 10 ml of pure alcohol. If the drink is extra-strength alcohol it is likely to count as two units.

What is often overlooked is how much weight drinking a lot regularly can put on. On Drinkaware's website you can find out exactly how much alcohol is in your favourite drink. It's a good idea to cut down on alcohol as part of a calorie-controlled diet and see how much difference it makes. See Further information on page 138.

You are what you eat – reasons for weight gain

There may be medical reasons for gaining weight, and if these are serious it is most likely that you are already seeing a doctor about them. However, other health issues can be resolved by changing what you eat and ditching the foods that are causing you to be overweight and unhealthy.

Blood sugar levels

Fast-releasing carbohydrates and fizzy drinks which are very high in sugar cause fluctuating blood sugar levels, giving 'highs' and 'lows' which become a vicious circle. Anyone who's ever felt a burst of energy after a sugary snack or drink followed by a slump in energy later on, will be aware of the ups and downs of fluctuating blood sugar levels. Sugary snacks and drinks increase weight, affect our blood sugar levels and have led to an epidemic of type II diabetes.

Stimulants such as tea and coffee, which contain caffeine, alcohol and refined carbohydrates – sugar, white bread, white rice, cereals, cakes, biscuits and chocolate all contribute to fluctuating blood sugar levels. And so does stress, which among other actions prompts the release of excess glucose into the blood.

Skipping meals is also likely to make blood sugar levels dip too low and can have the effect of increasing weight. Author Barbara Cousins, who wrote *Easy Tasty Healthy* and the *Cooking Without* series, explains, 'When blood sugar levels dip the metabolism slows down and there isn't enough energy to burn food so weight increases.' She recommends eating little and often – up to six meals a day of healthy foods.

All is not lost. By changing to healthy eating and drinking habits, blood sugar can be stabilised. This means that it becomes easier to lose weight and crucially the body is more energetic, which is a huge benefit.

Too much salt

Eating a diet that is high in salt makes the body retain fluid, a common problem in overweight people. It is also linked to high blood pressure and cardiovascular disease.[6] Salt is in many of the products we buy so it is worth checking the ingredients before purchase, and not adding salt in cooking or to meals.

There are some healthier salts, such as Himalayan crystal salt, which also contains trace minerals such as calcium and magnesium, or Herbamare which has added herbs.

It's important to flush toxins (including excess salt) out of the kidneys by drinking about eight glasses (2 litres) of water or herbal tea a day. However, green tea, dandelion and hibiscus herbal teas are diuretics, which increase the excretion of urine.

Allergies, intolerances and deficiencies

Our bodies are very clever and automatically surround alien substances with fluid, which causes fluid retention, which may or may not be obvious. A nutritional therapist automatically tests for allergies and intolerances, the most common of which are dairy and wheat. If visiting a nutritionist is too expensive, it is a good idea to cut out certain foods or drinks for a month or so to see if there is a difference in weight and/or wellbeing.

Nutritional experts can also discover if nutrients are not being properly absorbed, which can result in feeling hungry all the time and wanting to eat more.

There has been a huge rise in the number of people aware that they are intolerant of gluten and currently 8.5 million[7] in the UK are eating gluten-free diets. There is a big difference between being intolerant of gluten and the 1 per cent of people who are coeliac, an auto-immune disease that means the body cannot process gluten at all and has a very strong reaction to it.

There are anecdotal reports of people finding that their osteoarthritis improved when they gave up gluten. All UK supermarkets have 'Free From' sections where there are a variety of products without gluten in them. Your doctor can give you a test to see if you should be eating gluten-free foods, but even if you don't have to you can try cutting down the amount you eat and see if arthritic symptoms improve.

Cultivating friendly bacteria

In recent years there has been much talk about 'friendly' bacteria, and the health of the gut (from the mouth to the anus) has been highlighted as being essential to our overall health because it accounts for 70 per cent of our immune system. The bacteria in the large intestine are like a wild garden (known as the microbiome) with hundreds of different species, weighing around 2 kg (4-5 lb). In a healthy person the 'friendly' microflora cling to the wall of the large intestine like barnacles preventing harmful bacteria getting a hold on the surface.

However, they are constantly under attack from hostile bacteria, such as *E. coli* and *C. difficile* which become prevalent in the gut when we suffer from stress, take antibiotics, eat poorly, become ill, travel abroad, or drink too much alcohol.

Nutritionists often advocate taking probiotics to maintain the right balance of bacteria in the microbiome and for overall health. There is research going on all the time into the relationship between osteoarthritis and the health of the microbiome, and whether probiotics can help to ease its symptoms (see Chapter 7).

There are a few branded yoghurt drinks that have a concentrated dose of healthy bacteria in them, and some people find that these help their digestive system. Check ingredients for sugar levels which can make these drinks counter-productive.

Keeping a healthy microbiome can also prevent candida, a yeast infection which takes hold in the gut and seeps into the bloodstream causing various symptoms such as weight gain, digestive problems, athlete's foot and thrush. Doctors can prescribe antifungals, and there are specific herbal remedies and supplements available over the counter. Detoxifying from candida can be quite debilitating, with upset stomachs and headaches quite likely so it is better to be guided by a nutritionist or other medical expert.

Stress and pollution

The reason for eating healthy food, as in the Mediterranean diet, is to get a huge range of nutrients – vitamins and minerals. Unless you visit a nutritionist it is difficult to find out if you have any deficiencies in these, but it is generally understood that with today's polluted environment and intensive farming, which depletes the soil of essential minerals, it is hard to get all the nutrients we need. Nutritionists can also discover if nutrients are not being properly absorbed which can lead people to eat more because they feel hungry.

You can ask for a vitamin D test at the doctors, but unless you have specific conditions, they are unlikely to give you a full test for vitamins and minerals. See Further informationon on page 132 for details of tests.

Our insides face a whole host of chemicals which are in the air that we breathe, in the cleaning products used in the home, and in much of the food that we eat. If possible, it is better to eat organic food which has been grown in fields where harsh pesticides are not being used. Meat from organically reared animals does not contain growth hormones and antibiotics, which are not good for our health and can result in extra weight gain.

Detoxifying the body

Either with a nutritional therapist or by following a book on the subject (see page 137) it is possible to detoxify by cutting out saturated fat, sugar, salt, alcohol and processed foods – foods that are made in a factory. Nutritionists recommend detoxing with a diet high in vegetables and fruit (preferably organic), wholegrains such as brown rice and wholemeal bread, and pulses – including lentils and split peas.

This needs to be done gradually and with caution, especially if there is not a professional advisor helping. Dramatically changing what you eat in the long term leads to better health and weight control, but as the body adjusts and detoxifies, it's normal to feel unwell – maybe headaches and stomach pains can result and sometimes an overwhelming feeling of fatigue. As people progress with detoxifying it's also possible that deep seated emotions start to be released.

Meat and fish

Meat eaters should try to have more chicken and turkey than red meat and to choose organic so there are no traces of antibiotics, growth hormones or pesticides. There is often controversy about fish from the sea being polluted and farmed fish being subjected to toxic chemicals and causing environmental problems. Most people believe the benefits outweigh these problems, but if possible, it is better to choose organically farmed or wild salmon – it's much less pink because it hasn't been dyed!

Why is organic good?

Organic produce and meat can be more expensive than non-organic, but where possible if you can afford to buy it, it is preferable not to have traces of pesticides in your food whatever your state of health is. Some fruit and vegetables are sprayed many times with pesticides, and animals reared for meat are often routinely prescribed antibiotics and other drugs – organic meat farming does not allow routine prescription.

Chapter 6

Food and drink –
acidic or alkaline?

In healthcare people are often treated alike, but in reality, people are individuals and so are their bodies and health issues. Certain acidic foods can aggravate osteoarthritis in some people, but not necessarily everyone.

It is very simple to test your own acidity by buying some pH test strips from the pharmacist. These involve testing either your urine or saliva to get a reading but it is better not to do this straight after a meal as it may affect the result. If your acidity is very high you should certainly see a doctor, but if it is just a bit high there are various things you can do such as eating different sorts of foods, taking probiotics, or trying a balancing drink of aloe vera, or taking cider vinegar in water to lower acidity.

Food is such a pleasure to a lot of people that the thought of giving up certain foods can be distressing, but to stay one step ahead of osteoarthritis it is worth trying to exclude some foods for a while.

Diet, like exercise, is one of the keys to good health and after persisting with eliminating some of the foods you normally eat for a few weeks, it's quite common to start enjoying different foods and a healthy way of eating. There's nothing more encouraging than feeling good.

Acid versus alkaline

Some foods are reputed to aggravate arthritis because they are very acidic, and acid in the body aggravates osteoarthritis and other diseases. They may trigger inflammation and pain in some people but not in others.

Cutting out some acidic foods and bringing into your daily routine more alkaline foods, specifically vegetables, can make a big difference to how you cope with and prevent arthritis. Many elderly people with osteoarthritis have spent a lifetime eating a lot of potatoes and tomatoes and find the idea of giving them up depressing. If you exclude them for a short while, see if it makes a difference to symptoms – have the pain and inflammation eased? If the answer is yes, then you may need to have them only as special treats now and then or try some alternatives.

Medical herbalist Chris Etheridge suggests trying your own exclusion diet, cutting out dairy, wheat or meat or some of the foods on the following list to see if you have pain relief and reduced inflammation. All of these foods are acid-forming and so adopting a vegan diet could be helpful – but this is an unlikely choice for many older people.

Foods that could cause problems:

- Tomatoes, potatoes, aubergines, peppers – all plants in the 'nightshade' family have a reputation for aggravating osteoarthritis. Once again, by trial and error you can discover if this is true for you by excluding them for a month or more.
- Lemon juice is naturally acidic, but when it is fully metabolised in the body, and its minerals dissociated in the bloodstream, the effect is alkalising, and it raises the pH of body tissue. However, citrus fruit in general can affect some people with osteoarthritis, so once again try cutting down on these and see if it makes a difference.

- All meat is acid-forming.
- All wine is acidic, so it is preferable to drink very little or none at all. Again, see if this makes a difference.

Suggestions for alternative foods:
- Substitute sweet potatoes for potatoes – they are high in vitamins.
- Or instead of mashed potato, mash a mixture of other root vegetables, such as swede, carrots and turnips, which are all alkaline and nutritious.
- Nearly all vegetables are alkaline but be aware asparagus and Brussels sprouts are not.

As previously mentioned, nowadays, so many people have food intolerances and allergies that there is a 'Free From' section in every supermarket.

Foods that are good for osteoarthritis:
- A healthy diet packed with vegetables, brown rice, pulses, vegetable juices, oily fish and chicken, helps the body eliminate toxins.
- Turmeric, ginger (considered warming in Chinese medicine), olives, olive oil, green tea and grapes, all have a reputation for being good for arthritis.
- Alkaline foods such as avocados, spinach, radishes, beetroot, carrots, spinach, rhubarb, dried fruit and many fresh fruits are also good.

Barbara Cousins, nutritionist and author of *Easy, Tasty, Healthy* makes the point 'With both osteoarthritis and rheumatoid arthritis people are often allergic to dairy foods and wheat and need to cut these out. It is also important to avoid red meat because of its high acidity, as well as citrus fruit, and members of the nightshade family, such as potatoes, peppers, tomatoes and aubergines as most arthritis sufferers have an intolerance to them.

'To get the overload of toxins out of the body I put arthritis patients on a detoxification diet of vegetables, wholegrains such as brown rice, millet, quinoa and buckwheat, and lots of pulses – lentils and beans – while avoiding sugar and alcohol. Eating these foods supports the liver and bowel so that they can eliminate the toxins and stabilise blood sugar levels to give the internal organs more energy.

'People should start to notice improvements within a month, but it could take a year or more to really get on top of things, depending on the severity of the condition.'
(See Further information on page 135.)

Dehydration

Drinking plenty of water keeps the body hydrated. Chris Etheridge, medical herbalist, believes that a large percentage of the population is dehydrated, which is damaging to health in general. He says, 'When someone is dehydrated, inflammation increases. I recommend drinking 1.5 to 2 litres (2½ to 3 ½ pints) per day of fluids, and that includes tea and coffee.'

He warns against drinking fizzy drinks. 'They contain phosphoric acid, sugar and caffeine and leave people dehydrated, particularly in hot temperatures.' The problem with an abundance of phosphoric acid is that it strips calcium from the body.

What is particularly good and tasty are vegetable juices, home-made with a juicer, or a good quality ready-made juice available in health food stores and supermarkets (see Chapter 12).

Herbal teas contain no caffeine, and some contain herbs that are helpful for osteoarthritis, such as ginger which is warming and improves circulation. Nettle tea is also recommended as a cleanser, and for reducing pain and inflammation. If you don't like the taste you can mix it with peppermint or buy a tea that combines one or more herbs with nettle. Green tea contains less caffeine than black tea and is a good alternative as it has a lot of additional health benefits.

Does cider vinegar work?

Cider vinegar is often recommended as something to reduce the pain of arthritis, but does it work? It's cheap and easy to take cider vinegar in water every day, but a lot of people aren't too keen on it because of the acidic taste. While it seems counter-intuitive to have an acidic drink, the way it works is that the body metabolises cider vinegar, and it turns alkaline.

Apple cider vinegar 'with the Mother' means that it has not been pasteurised, contains a lot of beneficial bacteria, and is rich in minerals. It is easier to find this in a health store than a supermarket, and the good news is it's incredibly cheap – from around £3 for 750 ml (about 1⅓ pint).

The way to take it is to pour one dessertspoonful of cider vinegar 'with the Mother' into a glass of water (warm or cold) every morning or before all meals, if required. If you find it difficult to swallow you can start with a teaspoonful in water and gradually increase it or try adding a teaspoonful of honey to it. Good quality honey, particularly made by your local bees, contains trace elements of vitamins and minerals and, as it is made from the nectar of plants, is rich in plant compounds and antioxidants which fight free radicals that damage cells in the body.

The Margaret Hills programme

Apple cider vinegar is one of the main components of the approach developed by the Margaret Hills Clinic in Warwickshire, which has helped thousands of people with rheumatoid and osteoarthritis (among other conditions) with nutritional therapy. Now run by Margaret Hills' daughter, Christine Horner, the clinic's programme is based on apple cider vinegar with honey, molasses and Epsom salts baths. Margaret Hills claims that apple cider vinegar has the power to dissolve acid deposits in the joints and expel them through the kidneys.

The programme also comprises a strict acid-free diet, which includes cutting out a wide range of foods, including beef and pork, dairy products, citric acid-forming fruits, alcohol, tea, coffee, sugary and fizzy drinks, refined sugar, wheat and hot spices.

The diet focuses on eating plenty of vegetables, cooked and raw, brown rice and grains, fish, avocados, nuts and seeds and products made from them, and most herbs and spices. People following the programme are advised to take Margaret Hills supplements too.

It's a very strict regime, but many people have followed it independently or under supervision from the clinic, including Terence Jacques.

Case study: Terence Jacques, 80

In 2014, without warning at the age of 75, I suddenly developed severe pains in my left knee. After a GP visit and an X-ray I was diagnosed with the onset of osteoarthritis and was told it was age related. My GP told me the condition was chronic and irreversible. He told me the treatment was painkillers then stronger painkillers, followed by, if necessary, injections into my knee, and ultimately an operation using keyhole surgery. I told him I did not want any of these options and he repeated that the condition was irreversible.

I had read that a change of diet had helped people with osteoarthritis. I also recalled a good friend telling me years earlier that a change of diet had improved her arthritis. I asked the GP for his views on diet change. He replied that in all of his experience as a doctor there was no evidence whatsoever that diet could cure arthritis. He said this suggestion was entirely anecdotal with no medical evidence to support it.

However, I did not want to spend the rest of my life on painkillers which was the prognosis of my GP. Also, as I enjoy walking with the Ramblers, I decided to research diet as a viable option, and purchased a book by Margaret Hills. Eventually I also paid for a private online consultation which was well worth the money. (See Further information on page 130.)

Because the suggested diet change seemed highly plausible and a much more attractive option than what the NHS had to offer, I followed the advice with quick and remarkable results. Within five months I had no pain whatsoever, and after eight months the stiffness in my knee had also gone. It is now over five years later, and I am still entirely free from the crippling pain caused by arthritis.

In light of this experience, I am convinced much time and NHS money is wasted on unnecessary painkillers, injections and operations insofar as doctors seem reluctant to accept there are cheaper and more natural and effective alternatives.

I do tell friends and acquaintances who have arthritis they may want to give the Margaret Hills solution a try, as it worked for me. I lead walks for the Ramblers and do circuit training three times each week and am pain-free. I do point out that changing one's diet is, of course, not easy – far from it. But with determination and time, they will adjust, be healthier and arthritis free.

Chapter 7

Supplements and herbal medicine

Speak to someone about osteoarthritis and they will most likely tell you about the supplement they take and how good it is. The truth is that some work for some people and not for others – as, unsurprisingly, we are all different.

The supplements specifically recommended for osteoarthritis are not essential for the body, but can provide extra nutrition to help nourish joints, ease inflammation or reduce pain. Some more general supplements (such as vitamin C or vitamin B3) have many other actions to improve general health, including reducing inflammation and pain.

As a consumer you can get overwhelmed and confused – should you be taking minerals such as zinc, magnesium or calcium, and what do you choose? The work is done for you if you take a multivitamin/mineral so that you get the essential vitamins and minerals in one capsule/tablet. Similarly, it's worth looking at joint complexes which are very good for people with osteoarthritis and enable you to buy less but get everything you need.

Many people believe that they can get all the nutrients they need from their food, but unless you are tested by a nutritionist or doctor you do not know what deficiencies you have. Because supplements contain a concentrated amount of the vitamin, mineral or herb it is unlikely that you could eat anywhere near that amount on a day-to-day basis.

It is beyond the scope of this book to make specific recommendations about which supplements osteoarthritis sufferers should be taking, but a good multi-vitamin and multi-mineral are helpful for us all as we get older.

It is important to choose good quality supplements as some of the cheaper bulk-buy versions either don't contain enough of the active ingredient to be effective or may contain a number of 'fillers' which are just there to bulk out the tablet. So, it's worth spending a bit of time comparing the amount of active ingredients versus the prices and see if a good deal really is what it seems.

There are plenty of reputable manufacturers whose supplements are often vegan/vegetarian and don't contain extras that you don't need or want. See Further information on pages 135-137.

Health food stores are a great place to find out and buy good quality supplements. The staff are usually very knowledgeable and can help you with your queries.

Case study: My supplement list

Having tried all the supplements, I have finally found a combination that works for me: taken every morning on an empty stomach:

- Omega-3 fish oils: 2 x 1000 mg capsules

- Turmeric capsules: 1 or 2 x 620 mg capsules

- No blush niacinamide: 1 x 1000 mg x vitamin B3 in the morning with breakfast (+ one at lunch or dinner)

- Multivitamin/mineral: 1 a day

- Vitamin D 3000 IU spray: one spray under the tongue daily

- Vitamin C cherry liquid.

After six months of taking these and cutting out the most acidic foods, my fingers straightened out, were less swollen and were not giving me nearly so much pain. My knee is good enough for me to play tennis and live normally – apart from avoiding steep inclines downwards (see Chapter 2).

Popular osteoarthritis supplements

Dr Rod Hughes says, 'There is some strong evidence that supplements may help pain and stiffness in osteoarthritis. The evidence is best for daily GOPO® (rosehip – see page 69), omega-3 fish oils which may help pain, and glucosamine[1] which may slow down progress of osteoarthritis. Patients can try a variety of dietary changes to help arthritis but say that there is little evidence that the exclusion or inclusion of certain foods helps arthritis. Obviously, calorie restriction may help weight loss.'

- **Turmeric** has been used in Ayurvedic medicine for thousands of years and is particularly recommended for easing inflammation in osteoarthritis.[2] It is the curcumin in the root of the turmeric plant which has anti-inflammatory, antibacterial, antiviral and antifungal properties, and research is usually into curcumin, not into turmeric itself. When choosing a turmeric supplement make sure that the manufacturing process has enabled the curcumin to be released. This is achieved by heating up the turmeric root in oil or extracting it with alcohol and adding black pepper to increase its absorption in the body. Check the ingredients to see the level of curcuminoids and ask in the health food store if you need help. For ideas on how to take turmeric, see Chapter 12.

- **Fenugreek** seeds are rich in linolenic acids and have anti-inflammatory and anti-arthritic actions. Research has not been carried out on humans, but this is a spice you can add to cooking, and it is also available in capsule form.

- **Glucosamine**** is believed to rebuild cartilage, repair damage and relieve pain.

- **MSM** (mineral sulphur) is often combined with glucosamine to provide pain relief as arthritis sufferers may have a deficiency of sulphur. It is claimed that it may take some time for the effects to be felt.

- **Chondoitrin**** is often combined with glucosamine, because it attracts fluid into the cartilage which should make joints more mobile.
- **Rosehip**: GOPO® is a naturally occurring anti-inflammatory agent isolated from the seeds and husks of fruit (rosehips) from a sub-species of *Rosa canina* (dog-rose). Scientists have found that GOPO® can prevent the migration of inflammatory cells thought to be involved in triggering and maintaining joint inflammation.[3, 4, 5]
- **Hyaluronic acid** may be available in tablet form or injected into the joint, but the results are not definitive.

**Check the sources of these supplements – I tend to avoid anything from 'bovine' sources. Also, you need to look out for the inclusion of shellfish if you are allergic to it.

For people who prefer not to have supplements that are from animal sources, try a vegan/vegetarian alternative. The best way to find out is to look for the words 'vegetarian' and/or 'vegan' on the label – if it doesn't say, it's less likely that they are. Or you can look on the manufacturer's website for the full ingredients.

Vitamins, minerals and supplements

Dr Rod Hughes is convinced of the importance of vitamin D: 'About 50 per cent of the population is deficient in vitamin D, due to lack of exposure to the sun. Deficiency can mimic arthritis, providing the same symptoms. It's very easy to take a blood test and treatment is simple with capsules or injections, and the patient gets better very quickly.' One way to take vitamin D is in a simple-to-use spray in the mouth. See Further information on page 137.

- **Multivitamins**: The good thing about multivitamins/minerals is that you know that you are getting a complete spread of all the vital vitamins and minerals. Unless you visit a nutritionist and are tested for deficiencies, you do not know what your status is.

- **Vitamin B3 (niacin/niacinamide)**: Patrick Holford in his book, *Say No to Arthritis*,[6] gives a compelling history of the efficacy of vitamin B3 in reducing inflammation and making joints more mobile. It's important to buy niacinamide or no-blush/flush niacin because the standard niacin can bring on a strange blushing sensation.

- **Vitamin C**: Most of us think of vitamin C as helping us to ward off colds and flu, but it has many other actions in the body. It has been found in research to be effective in reducing inflammation in osteoarthritis and impeding its progress.[7] Taking high amounts of vitamin C cannot harm you as excess is excreted out of the body, though at a very high level it can give you diarrhoea.

- **Vitamin D**: The body makes vitamin D when skin is exposed to the sun, which means people who cover up do not get enough sun rays. Also found in oily fish, eggs, dairy products, green leafy vegetables and mushrooms, it is required for healthy bones and teeth and good muscle function.[8]

- **Omega-3 fish oils** reduce inflammation and increase mobility. There are two types of omega-3 fatty acids: DHA (docosahexaenoic acid) and EPA (eicosapentaenoic acid). Researchers have found that EPA and DHA both reduce inflammation.[9] There are vegetarian and vegan alternatives.

- **Magnesium** among other vital functions relaxes muscles, and can ease aches and pains. Magnesium oil sprays are an easy way to soothe muscles after activity.[10] Magnesium works with calcium and phosphorus to maintain healthy bones in older age.

- **Probiotics** are considered by nutritionists to be one of the most important supplements you can take. As most people must know from TV commercials probiotics ensure that the gut (which runs from the mouth to the anus) is populated with healthy bacteria (microflora). The health of the gastro-intestinal tract accounts for 70 per cent of the health of our immune system, so by keeping it healthy we stand a better chance of maintaining our wellbeing. Scientists are constantly finding more out about how the body works and are looking at the link between the microbiome, obesity and osteoarthritis.

- **Aloe vera**: is alkaline and helps to counter acidity in the body and also has anti-inflammatory properties. It is available as a liquid in bottles and although it's not a great taste, you can mix it with juice or drink a small amount or take capsules if you can't bear the flavour.

See Further information on pages 135-137 for more details of supplements and recommendations. There are always vegetarian/vegan options too.

Herbal medicine

Medical herbalist, Chris Etheridge, advocates a body-wide treatment plan for his patients, which includes gentle exercise, healthy eating and providing herbal remedies that are anti-inflammatory and therefore reduce swelling around the joint and ease pain.

A session with a medical herbalist like Chris involves an initial consultation in which he asks about past medical history, whether or not the patient has taken drugs in the past, family and social history, and how the whole body is working. 'I ask them if they have ever done any heavy lifting or digging because it has an impact on wear and tear.'

One reason for taking herbal remedies is that some people prefer more natural treatments than painkillers or non-steroidal anti-inflammatory drugs, such as ibuprofen, which can cause gastric problems if taken long term.

Warning: The herbalist will ask if you are on any medications in case herbal remedies interact with them, but if you are buying over-the-counter remedies it is important to find out whether you can take them with various pharmaceutical drugs.

Pain relief

Chris Etheridge explains, 'Turmeric and ginger, meadowsweet, willow, birch and poplar, all contain chemicals that work in a similar way to how aspirin and other anti-inflammatories are known to act.'

- **White willow** contains salicylic acid (which is also in aspirin) and is anti-inflammatory and pain relieving.
- **Devil's claw** (*Harpagophytum*) is widely used in Europe (where herbal medicine is much more accepted than in the UK) as a natural anti-inflammatory for arthritis. It doesn't have many side-effects and is considered to be safe.
- **Stinging nettle** is often used in teas and is believed to cleanse the system. A trial using stinging nettle leaves directly on osteoarthritic thumbs showed a reduction of pain when compared with a placebo.[11]
- **Turmeric** (already described under supplements) may also be suggested by a medical herbalist. Supplements provide just the right amount of turmeric, containing the essential curcumin ingredient, but cooking with turmeric is also beneficial for osteoarthritis (see Chapter 12).
- **Ginger** is an anti-inflammatory and warming to the system. It can be eaten in food, taken as a supplement, in a tincture or as a home-made or shop-bought tea. It can also be grated into hot water in a bowl for soaking hands or feet to ease inflammation and pain.
- **Capsicum cream** (chilli) for nerve pain is both anti-inflammatory and pain relieving when rubbed on joints.
- **Boswellia** (also known as Indian frankincense) is believed

to have anti-inflammatory and pain-relieving properties,[12] and is widely used in Ayurvedic medicine (see later in this chapter, page 76).

- **Arnica**: Arnica gel is a herbal preparation which has an anti-inflammatory effect, not to be confused with the homeopathic Arnica tablets for bruising which are derived from the same plant but prepared differently. In a study of people with osteoarthritis of at least one knee joint, rubbing Arnica gel on the joint(s) twice daily gave them significant treatment success after just three weeks. The inflammatory pain diminished considerably.[13] In a study conducted on more than 200 people with osteoarthritic pain in the fingers, Arnica gel was shown to be as effective as ibuprofen gel, with patients generally preferring Arnica gel to the synthetic gel. The number of painful joints was decreased significantly, and morning joint stiffness decreased.[14]

- **Comfrey root** used externally in a cream or in oil, has been shown to be effective in reducing inflammation and pain in osteoarthritis. It has been used for hundreds of years and is mentioned in Shakespeare's plays. Several recent randomised clinical trials substantiate the efficacy of topical comfrey preparations in the treatment of pain, inflammation and swelling of muscles and joints in the case of degenerative arthritis.[15]

- **Meadowsweet** contains aspirin-like compounds for pain relief. It was also used hundreds of years ago and is cited in Shakespeare's plays.

- **Cannabis oil (CBD or cannabidiol)** has recently become available in health stores. It doesn't contain the hallucinogenic component of cannabis but does help with pain. For years people have been smoking or eating the drug to ease pain, but this way it is in a spray or lotion which is now legal! Recent studies show that CBD oil (cannabidiol), which is extracted from the cannabis plant, may alleviate pain and inflammation in diseases such as osteoarthritis.[16]

Bee venom – an old wives' tale?

It has been said that bee venom can be very good for soothing osteoarthritis, but while research is currently being conducted it is not yet conclusive. So, here is a funny story.

Case study: Kathi

French teacher, Kathi, decided to stop travelling so far to lessons because she was suffering from osteoarthritis in her hands which was uncomfortable and painful. She tells the story, 'I was at the top of the garden, clearing scrub and must have uncovered a mining bee nest. As I was finishing off a large bee flew up to me and seemed to look at me, then appeared to consciously choose to sting my left knuckle.

The area swelled up and I applied some antihistamine cream to it on the pharmacist's advice. A week later it started swelling up again to the point that I could barely use the hand. I don't remember it being particularly itchy, but it was warm to the touch. Back to the chemist's and I took some stronger oral antihistamine after that.

I'd been having discomfort and sometimes pain in my finger joints for a few months, especially after any prolonged use. After the reaction to the sting had abated, I didn't feel any pain for a couple of months and I hardly feel more than passing discomfort at the moment, several months later. I had an X-ray and am supposed to go back to see a rheumatologist at some stage if after another blood test results aren't great. I've been lax about doing this as I feel a fraud, as I barely feel joint pain now, just discomfort! Bless the bees!'

Creams and oils

There are a number of all-in-one oils or lotions that can help with joint pain and these include:

- **Castor oil**: Older readers may remember their grannies or mums using castor oil when they were young. Sometimes it was used internally as a laxative, but its anti-inflammatory properties are just as valid now as they were back then. It's a relatively cheap oil to buy and you can rub it into a swollen joint to relieve swelling and pain.
- **Chinese Wood Lock oil** (methyl salicylate 50 per cent, menthol 16 per cent, camphor 10 per cent) is very strong but eases pain.
- **Tiger Balm** (camphor, mint oil, cajuput oil, menthol and clove oil) has a similar effect to Chinese Wood Lock.
- **Pharmaceutical options** are ibuprofen-based, such as Voltarol and Nurofen Gel, but too much use of these can cause damage to the stomach lining and kidneys. Deep Freeze can also provide temporary relief for pain.

It is important to go to a registered medical herbalist, not someone who has just set up and doesn't appear to be affiliated to an official body. Go to Further information on page 131 for details of how to find one.

Chinese herbal medicine

Make sure that you choose a bona fide practitioner who is affiliated to the main association (see Further information, page 128). Chinese herbal medicine is well established in the UK.

The principles of Chinese medicine are based on the meridians or channels running through the body that carry *qi* or *chi* or energy. It is along these meridians that practitioners put acupuncture needles and use acupressure (see Chapter 8).

The doctor looks at the patient's tongue and takes their pulse – there are 12 pulses in Chinese medicine, and these indicate where energy is weak. Herbs are chosen according to whether symptoms indicate damp, heat, or cold in the body, and the aim is to unblock stagnant energy.

Ayurvedic medicine

Evolved over thousands of years in India and the Asian continent, Ayurveda comprises yoga, nutrition, herbal medicine, breathing and meditation. Everyone is treated individually according to which of three 'doshas' (constititutions) they are, which is established by observation, pulse reading and questioning.

Some of the Ayurvedic herbs that are helpful for osteoarthritis include *Boswellia serrata, Commiphora wightii, Astralagus,* turmeric and ginger,[17] says Dr Shijoe Mathew Anchery, an Ayurvedic doctor who used to work at the Ananda Spa, in the Himalayas (see Further information, page 129). Dr Anchery comments:

'In Ayurvedic medicine we want to find out where the osteoarthritis is coming from – age, wear and tear or an imbalance in the body. For instance, a *dosha* imbalance may manifest primarily as dryness in the body – such as dry eyes, dry mouth, or constipation, clicking and creaking sounds in joints, which would eventually lead to a degenerative joint condition.'

Dr Anchery explains that oils can be used both externally and internally to lubricate the body – ghee oil, olive oil, sesame oil (and sesame seeds) are particularly good for taking internally. 'Oil pooling treatment in Ayurveda is when you create a reservoir around a joint – such as in the hollow in the back of the neck or the knee where you put warm, medicated oil and leave it there to soak in.

'Osteoarthritis can result from digestive issues – where people are often bloated, and not absorbing nutrients properly. Or it can be due to a heat imbalance in the body which is often aggravated by hormonal problems. Alternatively, for other people it could be due to cold and damp exposure – people who feel cold in the extremities, and who forget to drink water because they feel cold, causing more dryness. The remedies recommended for each of these causative factors will be different in Ayurveda based on its actual root cause. So, digestion has to improve for one person, and for another oil and warm food are sufficient'.

Chapter 8

Therapies to manage pain

Looking after your body means attending to problems as and when they appear – this means that niggling backaches and pains in the legs, shoulders or arms may benefit from massage or some adjustments, but they don't always require drugs. It is wise to go to a physiotherapist, chiropractor, or osteopath when you have pain or other problems involving your joints/movement.

Physiotherapy

Osteoarthritis is a slow, degenerative disease, and so there may be early signs that cause no problem at all. 'Some people may have a bit of a knee problem, for instance, that bothers them some of the time, but not always,' says Sammy Margo, chartered physiotherapist. 'Others may have a more acute joint that is painful but does not interfere with their normal life. At the chronic stage, arthritis is disabling and joints can become deformed.'

Physiotherapists use a range of different methods including mobilisation of the joint through massage and manipulation, electrotherapy (ultrasound or TENS), acupuncture, strengthening and stretching limbs, and balance work.

Sammy Margo says, 'We want people to be empowered, so that they can go away and be able to cope if they have a flare up.

If they keep on doing the same things, they won't get any better.

'We look at their core stability to see if their tummy and buttock muscles are weak and not supporting them well. We also look at the way they walk and see if there are changes they can make to put less pressure on their lower body.'

'There is plenty of self-management that people can do – for instance, icing the joint when it flares up, helps to bring down swelling – but they also need to look at their lifestyle, including sedentary job effects, weight loss, and what shoes they wear. High heels put huge stress on your feet and your knees, increasing the chances of getting osteoarthritis.'

If you are in the UK, your doctor can refer you to a physiotherapist on the NHS if s/he thinks it will help. In theory you should be able to go to a chiropractor or osteopath on the NHS, but in practice, this doesn't happen very often. It is worth asking the GP about this, as Clinical Commissioning Groups (CCGs) vary as to what they can provide.

Chiropractic and osteopathy

Having regular treatments with a chiropractor or osteopath helps to keep your body fit and prevent pain (including the pain of arthritis). You can manage arthritis better if you take care of your body on a regular basis, instead of thinking 'it will just go away'.

Osteopathy and chiropractic are similar in the way that people are treated. Short thrusting movements are made with the hands to the spine in order to realign the vertebrae. The clicking sound is believed to be the release of a bubble of gas from the joint. Both osteopaths and chiropractors use a range of other treatments including massage to ease discomfort.

While osteopaths concentrate on the joints, tissues, muscles, ligaments and tendons, a chiropractor focuses on the musculoskeletal system – the bones, joints and muscles – and the effects of musculoskeletal disorders on the function of the nervous system and general health. For people who don't like the clicking, a McTimoney chiropractor uses a flicking motion which is light, fast and accurate.

It is worthwhile having misalignments corrected so as not to carry the problem around forever. After a lifetime with (say) headaches, neck pain or backache, when a misalignment that has been there for many years is released, it can take away the pain for the first time in years.

If you choose to go to a chiropractor or osteopath you will most likely have to pay for it unless you have health insurance. In most cases you can go as and when you need to and do not need to be tied into a course of treatment.

Acupuncture

Despite some people worrying about the idea of acupuncture because they don't like needles, it is nothing like an injection. The needles do not go in at a deep level and although it's possible to feel some of them, others are inserted without any sensation at all.

Acupuncture aims to increase energy (or 'chi') and blood flow through releasing energy blocks in the meridians – the channels believed in eastern medicine to run throughout the body.

A visit to an acupuncturist involves a lot of questions about wellbeing and how your body works as a whole. As it is a holistic treatment, the acupuncturist should establish underlying health patterns that relate to the osteoarthritis and any other conditions, so they don't just treat one thing but are aiming to free up areas of blocked 'chi' or energy and boost wellbeing. Needles are therefore placed in acupressure points around the inflamed joints and in other key points that relate to systemic health issues.

Acupuncture is a component of the system of Chinese medicine and has been widely used in Asia for thousands of years. It is now recognised by medical experts in the west and is sometimes available in NHS pain clinics within hospitals. Some GPs have been trained to provide acupuncture as an extra service for their patients.

Although it is one of the most recognised therapies in the UK, acupuncturists do vary in quality. If they ask a lot of questions and plan to treat you in a systemic way as well as locally, that is a good sign, but choosing a member of the British Council of Acupuncture ensures that you get a qualified practitioner.

There have been trials into the effectiveness of acupuncture for chronic pain[1] and it has been found to be one of the most effective physical treatments for osteoarthritis of the knee.[2]

Case study: Rob Philips

Rob Philips of North Devon fell over on the golf course and his thumbs flared up dramatically. 'I had suspected that I had osteoarthritis, but it wasn't until this happened that I found out for certain.'

Rob's doctor diagnosed tendonitis and put him on a regime of steroids. 'One night I was in so much pain that I went to A&E where they initially diagnosed a fracture, but subsequently realised it was osteoarthritis. I was prescribed six codeine-based painkillers a day, steroids, and due to the side-effects of the latter I had to have medication for my stomach. I also had steroid cream which made my hands red, inflamed and swollen in the sun because of the reaction to the UV rays.'

This was very inconvenient as Rob and his wife visit their daughter and family in Australia for a couple of months every year. Rob's wife was chatting to someone at the WI who suggested acupuncture might help. 'I have to say,' Rob continues, 'I am quite sceptical about these things, so I did a bit of local research and liked the idea of Alison Savory because she has a medical background.

'I wasn't worried about the needles at all, although sometimes the odd one is quite painful. I found Alison very bubbly and chatty and she told me, 'I can help you with all these things'.

I stopped using the steroid cream straight after the first session and gave up all the medication. This was due to the feeling of confidence that she would help me.

'Now after each session with Alison I feel great. I don't care *how* it has helped me – it could be psychosomatic to be honest – but I am now keeping on top of it. I can live with any underlying pain. There have been several by-products of having acupuncture – I have had asthma for 40 years and usually double the asthma spray doses in winter. This year I haven't needed to for the first time ever. Also, I had lots of liver spots on my back and they have started going since I've been to Alison.'

Alison Savory explains, 'The aim is to find the root cause of the problem and with arthritis we often look to digestion. It is quite common that when someone is taking medication, we have to work on alleviating the side-effects and gradually wean them off it. As they start to feel better, they decrease the medication, and eventually it is no longer needed. When someone has been taking steroids, the kidneys can become depleted. As the kidneys govern the bones in Chinese medicine, in the case of osteoarthritis, over time they can make a bad situation worse.

'Acupuncture is a powerful system of medicine that engages with the whole body. In the right hands it is very effective, but it is important that the acupuncturist is fully trained, as all members of the British Acupuncture Council are.'

Hyperbaric oxygen therapy

Athletes and sports people, such as footballers, tennis players and marathon runners, put enormous stress on their bodies and are more likely to get osteoarthritis in their joints because of this. Many have benefited from HBOT (hyperbaric oxygen therapy) which is helpful for a variety of conditions, including osteoarthritis.

It involves spending 50 minutes inside an oxygen chamber where the level of O_2 you receive is up to 97.7 per cent as opposed to the 21 per cent we all breathe in day to day.

The benefits for osteoarthritis are:

- Under pressure, HBOT acts as an anti-inflammatory,

removing swelling around joints by providing a good flow of oxygen around them. Normally, where there is swelling it prevents oxygen getting into the area.

- Red blood cells are increased. Because O_2 is a gas it dissolves into fluid under pressure and gets into the haemoglobin, lymph fluid and plasma.
- Increased levels of oxygen produce healing within the body, so that fractures and other injuries heal quicker.
- The white cell count goes up, which builds up the immune system, making the body more able to fight infection. Chronic osteoarthritic joints can become infected.
- It strengthens bones thereby producing more blood cells, as they are generated from the marrow in bones.

People are advised to go for 10 sessions of oxygen therapy if they have mild to moderate symptoms, and to go back every few months for a top up. For those people who have severe osteoarthritis, the number of sessions recommended is between 20 and 60.

Complementary therapies

Below are a few complementary therapies which can be helpful for osteoarthritis. Sometimes the effect of spending an hour or so dedicated to looking after yourself can be very relaxing, provide relief and make you feel good.

In most cases you have to pay for therapies, unless you have a local charity or organisation that provides them free. In the UK, cancer patients usually have access to therapies through Macmillan Cancer centres in hospitals.

- **Aromatherapy** involves full body, head, neck or back massage with essential oils. Essential oils are made from plants, trees and other natural sources and are believed to have therapeutic properties for both physical and emotional wellbeing. Rosemary and ginger oils are particularly good for arthritis and you can make up a blend in a carrier oil and rub it on painful areas yourself. As it is a massage treatment, aromatherapy helps to improve blood flow and circulation and provides relief for tight muscles.

- **Bowen technique**: is an alternative form of massage therapy that uses gentle touch to encourage the body to actively engage its own healing ability. It is applied using the fingers and thumbs to make small, rolling movements over muscles, tendons, ligaments and soft tissues at precise points on the body, using appropriate pressure for that individual. It can be very effective for areas of pain.

- **Herbal medicine**: While herbal remedies are available in health stores, it is often advisable to visit a registered medical herbalist. Properly qualified herbalists will have studied for three years full time and can give advice and prescribe herbal infusions for pain and inflammation (see Chapter 7).

- **Emmett technique** is a relatively new muscle release technique, devised by Ross Emmett. It is a gentle, safe and simple-to-apply muscle-release therapy. The therapist applies light finger pressure on specific parts of the body, which usually releases tension and pain, improves mobility and helps people to relax.

- **Homeopathy** is a gentle system of medicine which uses diluted extracts from plants and minerals available in a small sugar pill. They are completely safe for any age group, even if the recipient is on medication. The homeopath spends a long time taking details of a person's characteristics and likes and dislikes as well as their physical symptoms, and treats the person as a whole. The important thing that people don't always realise about homeopathy is that each person is treated as an individual. Ann-Louise Holland, a practising homeopath, explains, 'We treat the person, not the arthritis. Osteoarthritis can indicate rigidity in the body and may relate to past hurts and grief which have been held deep inside. The remedy addresses the emotional state of the person as well as the physical.'

- **Naturopathy** is a holistic approach to health care that incorporates nutrition, homeopathy and herbal medicine. The aim is to provide the right conditions for the body to heal itself, with particular focus on diet and lifestyle. Naturopaths place a lot of emphasis on emotional wellbeing and ask questions to establish whether or not the patient is in any kind of abusive relationship – not just with partners.
- **Reiki** is a form of healing which draws negative energy away from the body and helps you to relax. When you go to a healer you lie on a couch while they move around you, usually holding their hands just above you. It's very relaxing and can be helpful if you are in pain.
- **Massage**: Massaging the area where there is inflammation or pain can be very soothing. It also encourages blood flow, improves circulation and eases tension in muscles and tissues. There are different types of massage, and you can ask for the pressure to be gentle if you have a lot of pain. You can find a massage therapist at natural health shops and clinics, gyms, and beauty salons; many practitioners also work from home.
- **Reflexology**: A reflexologist massages or kneads the foot in a systematic way to stimulate parts of the body, which are reflected on the soles and sides of the feet. Areas that are particularly painful indicate that there is a weakness and so reflexology can be used for diagnosis. It's a thoroughly relaxing therapy as you can lie back and even fall asleep.

For details of associations and how to find therapists go to Further information on pages 128. For talking therapies, see Chapter 11.

Chapter 9

Practical ideas to make life easier

Modern life doesn't suit our bodies very well as, for example, sitting at computers and driving cars are not natural activities. Recent research has shown that our sedentary lifestyle could account for increasing levels of osteoarthritis.

Sedentary lifestyle research

Researchers at Harvard University in the US wanted to find out why osteoarthritis of the knee had doubled in the last 100 years. They examined skeletons in medical research facilities and museums in the States, and found that osteoarthritis of the knee was far less common in the past.[1]

- They inspected the skeletons of 1581 people who lived during the 19th century, and who were aged 50 or over, and compared them with those of 819 similar people who lived in the 20th century.
- After taking into account age and body mass index, cases of knee arthritis had doubled in the 20th century group – which suggests that something other than age and body weight had something to do with the increase.
- The researchers concluded that lifestyle was causing the problem – lack of exercise and sedentary jobs, diet and sports injuries. Another main culprit was likely to be

environmental factors, such as air pollution, as this was something that had dramatically increased in 100 years.

What you can do at work

Technology has revolutionised business and made it faster to complete work and communicate with people around the world. Conversely, it means that many more people sit down all day at a desk in front of a screen. This is taking its toll in many ways on our health, and if you have osteoarthritis you want to avoid sitting still for too long to prevent stiffness and pain.

Musculoskeletal disorders accounted for 35 per cent of self-reported illnesses according to the Health & Safety Executive (HSE) statistics for 'New and Long-standing Cases of Work Related Ill Health by Type, 2017/18'.[2] This was second to 'stress, depression or anxiety' which was at 44 per cent.

The campaign 'On Your Feet Britain'[3] makes the following suggestions for people who sit down for most of the day:

- stand during phone calls
- stand and take a break from your computer every 30 minutes
- use the stairs
- have standing or walking meetings
- eat your lunch away from your desk (or preferably go out for a stroll)
- walk to your colleagues' desks instead of phoning or emailing them
- stand at the back of the room during presentations.

For people who spend most of the day sitting at work, think carefully about the chair you are sitting in. Employers are not always helpful about providing comfortable and supportive chairs. If you can influence the type of chair there are some excellent choices that are ergonomically designed. To improve a not-so-good one, you may find that putting a rolled-up towel at the base of your spine makes a difference, or you can look at the numerous back support cushions available online.

A Backfriend (see page 139) is particularly good for supporting your whole back and keeping you in the right position when you're using a computer. Your feet should be flat on the floor and you should be close to the desk but not too close to the screen. Try to lean back from the computer into your chair rather than slumping forward peering at the screen – which most people seem to do. Clamping a phone with your neck is another habit which is all too common and will eventually result in neck and back problems.

Stand while you work

Even better than improving how you sit is standing for periods each day. Keeping active while at work is an easy way to keep your heart performing at its optimum level. A paper in *The British Journal of Sports Medicine* recommends that people in desk jobs should aim for at least two hours of standing a day.[4]

A standing or adjustable desk can be used at different levels, so that you can choose to sit for some of the time, and build up to a few hours' standing. While standing you are never still so your body remains slightly active and muscles and joints don't stiffen up.

The benefits of standing at your desk are:
- improved circulation
- lower blood pressure
- using up to 50 calories per hour.

The infographic opposite demonstrates how standing at work equates to running in terms of calories burned.

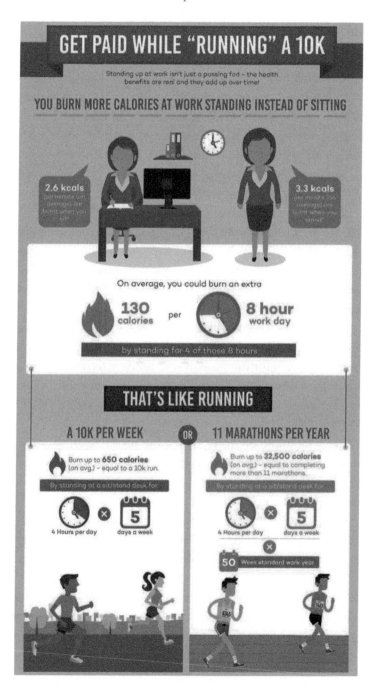

Look after your hands

What you do at the desk is important too – it's not just the sitting that is causing problems. We are overusing our hands when we type on keyboards and click the mouse. See if you can learn how to use the mouse on the other side – if you're right-handed, try using it with your left hand, and then swap back after a few weeks. It may help to try an ergonomic mouse, but whatever you use it involves repetitive use of your thumb and/or index finger.

Also, because of the way we sit we often cause extra strain on our backs, arms and hands.

As for texting and using tablets, the next generation are likely to have arthritic thumbs because of the amount of use they give them. Tablets may be a great invention, but sitting hunched over them is causing tight shoulders, back pain and neck ache as well as over-used hands.

All of us seem to need to use our fingers and thumbs more than we used to – texting on mobile phones, using iPads and other tablets, opening doors on the car. Modern technology takes little account of sore or swollen fingers and so many things have push buttons to operate them – remote controls, radio, TV, and so on.

The infographic opposite shows the alarming pressure we put on our fingers when using computers day in day out. Carpal tunnel syndrome is something that people with osteoarthritis in their hands certainly don't want.

When you see the amount of pressure that is put on hands using keyboards, it brings to mind the old manual typewriters where users had to bash down on the keys; this was really hard on the fingers.

Simply being aware of where and when you are putting strain on your body and hands helps. The Alexander Technique outlined in Chapter 4 (page 43) teaches us to become aware of where we are holding tension and causing unnecessary strain.

HOW MUCH PRESSURE ARE YOUR HANDS UNDER?

Repetitive typing and key entry is highly associated with Carpal Tunnel Syndrome. The typing speed may affect risk. For example typists whose speed is 60 words per minute exert up to 25 tons of pressure each day. It is also proven that typists with CTS struck the keys with greater force than those without the condition did.

40 words a minute

12,000 keys per hour

96,000 keys per 8-hour day

=

UP TO

25 TONS

8 ounces of force per key

16-25 tons of force each day

Speech recognition on computers is in the early stages and it would require a changed way of working, but it could save our fingers.

Wear supportive footwear

Of course, it's no good standing at work if you're wearing shoes that aren't comfortable. Not only would you end up with very tired feet, but high heels or uncomfortable shoes or boots can cause more discomfort in the body and be counter-productive.

Dr Roger Wolman, consultant rheumatologist at the Royal National Orthopaedic Hospital, points out, 'People should wear good cushioned shoes such as trainers or running shoes which are more efficient as shock absorbers, when the joints have lost their natural ability to do this.'

It's quite common to see young women commuting in their trainers and changing into their heels when they get to work. High heels are very popular with some women, but not only are they bad for your feet, they can cause back and leg pain. For anyone with osteoarthritis in the knees or hips they can exacerbate pain and inflammation and increase the likelihood of falling. See page 139 for recommendations of comfortable shoe manufacturers.

Carrying bags

Women have a particular problem with their handbags which are often bulky and heavy and put excessive pressure on hands, arms and shoulders. The easy solution is to start wearing a backpack or rucksack, some of which are now designed to look like handbags and are quite smart. Make sure the straps are adjusted to make it ultra-comfortable.

Benefits of rucksacks/backpacks include:
* they free up your hands

- your shoulders are pulled back and not hunched up
- the load is easier to carry on your back than on your hands, wrists, arms or one shoulder.

Shopping baskets at supermarkets are often quite heavy to lug around the store, so always choose a trolley. If you are in a car you can of course transport the goods directly to your boot without much lifting. If possible, ask someone stronger to carry the bags into the house on arrival at home.

If you don't drive and can't get someone to help you, you might prefer to order online which is possible at most supermarkets now, and have your groceries delivered to your doorstep.

Making the home a safe place

When you have osteoarthritis and you are getting older the last thing you want is to fall over. It is said that most accidents happen in the home, so it's sensible to identify and minimise hazards that you've been putting up with for years. There are simple things you can do to prevent accidents.

Kitchens, bathrooms and stairs

These are the most common places for accidents to happen, so, what can you do?

- Have the electric kettle near the tap if possible so that you don't have to walk across the room holding a heavy and/or hot kettle, putting pressure on arthritic hands.
- Rearrange the cupboards so that you're not bending and stretching inappropriately to get out everyday utensils or food.
- Invest in a non-slip bath/shower mat to help prevent slipping in the shower where water and soap/liquid soap can make it a dangerous place to be.

- Don't leave handbags, shoes, trailing wires or any other clutter on the floor where they are easy to trip over.
- Make sure the carpet on the stairs is tightly fitted so that it doesn't trip you up.
- If the stairs aren't carpeted, take extra care coming down them and don't wear socks which make it even more slippery.
- Wear shoes with soles rather than slippers (particularly those with no back) which can fall off and trip you up.

Dr Chris Steele, GP, and resident doctor on ITV's *This Morning*, sees plenty of people with osteoarthritis and says that it can cause a vicious circle, particularly among the elderly. 'Whenever I see a rug in an elderly person's house,' Chris says, 'I ask them to take it away, because they are so easy to trip over. People who cannot move easily tend to shuffle their feet, making them more likely to fall over and fracture bones. This is exacerbated by the number of older people with osteoporosis, which makes them more vulnerable to fractures.'

There is plenty of help about preventing falls on the NHS website. See Further information on page 126.

Household aids for the less mobile

For anyone who needs aids around the home, there is much that can be done – enquire at the local council and The Disabled Living Foundation. Grab rails, gates for the stairs and ramps can be installed and a whole range of gadgets for the kitchen can help people whose hands are arthritic. See Further information on page 125.

Chapter 10

The power of sleep and the weather

Few people realise the importance of a good night's sleep, but it is one of the pillars of good health. Our bodies are healing while we sleep so we need good restorative and regenerative sleep every night for around seven to eight hours. A good night makes you feel more energetic and ready for the day.

On the other hand, a bad night can make you feel terrible, and a string of sleepless or disturbed nights wears you down. Nothing feels right, your aches and pains are worse, and you can eventually become anxious and/or depressed. Continuous insomnia can lead to physical and mental health issues and exacerbate any health issues you already have.

As people get older they almost seem to accept that they won't sleep as well as they used to, but there are plenty of things that can help.

People have different patterns of sleeplessness:

- some find it hard to get to sleep
- others easily fall asleep but wake up in the early hours and have long periods of time lying awake
- others wake up very early in the morning and can't relax enough to get back to sleep
- and others wake up tired after what they thought was a good night; this may mean that sleep is not deep enough.

Self-help for insomnia

A word of warning: if insomnia is a new habit and you aren't worrying particularly about something specific, it is important to see your doctor to rule out any health problems.

Reasons for not sleeping well can include:

- stress and anxiety – worrying during the night
- being in pain or discomfort
- being too hot or too cold
- too much noise
- drinking caffeine or alcohol before bedtime
- over-stimulation before bed from watching TV or being on the internet
- going to bed too late for your body clock.

Ways in which you might improve your sleep include:

- Try to wind down before going to bed by listening to relaxing music, reading a book, or lying down and breathing deeply. Deep breathing is immensely calming for the mind and relaxing for the body.
- Avoid watching stimulating or frightening films or television programmes just before bedtime, particularly in the bedroom.
- You can find out if caffeinated drinks, such as coffee, tea or colas, are affecting you by cutting them out in the evening for a few weeks. Try decaffeinated coffee/tea, barley coffee substitutes, or herbal teas.
- If you drink alcohol, it's best to drink early in the evening, as it is dehydrating and may help you to fall asleep but wakes you up later on.
- Try a hot bath with a few drops of lavender essential oil dispersed in the water before bedtime. It also enables you to start the night off feeling warm.
- Some people swear by a nap in the day, but it can set up a vicious circle of not sleeping well at night and catching up

each day, so try to manage without and see if nights are better.

- A few drops of lavender essential oil on a tissue close to your face can be very soothing and sleep-inducing (and completely safe to use).
- There are a number of herbal and plant remedies which are safe to take and can ensure a better sleep. These include valerian, hops, and passiflora. If you are on medication, check with a doctor, pharmacist or the manufacturer (of herbal medicines) before taking herbal remedies. See Further information on page 131.
- Rescue Remedy is made up of flower essences and is unlikely to interact with medicines but check with a medical professional to be on the safe side. It can help to calm you during the day or night.
- Try using ear plugs if your partner snores.
- If light outside is a problem, you could change to darker or even black-out curtains or blinds.
- Some people find that it suits them to get up for a while in the middle of the night, rather than lying there counting sheep; do what works for you but don't get into a vicious circle.

Banishing electronic gadgets

Tech companies deny that their products affect our bodies, but if sleeping is a problem it is worthwhile considering the following points.

- Keep mobile and cordless phones either fully switched off during sleeping hours, or out of the bedroom.
- Don't use computer screens, tablets or phones just before bedtime – it has been shown that the blue light suppresses the production of melatonin, the hormone that induces sleep.

- Don't keep a clock with bright or flashing digits right by the bed. Try a traditional clock or move the digital one to the other side of the room. You can also often change the settings on digital clocks to reduce the brightness of the display.
- Keep televisions for the living rooms and switch off all lights/buttons in the bedroom.
- Don't have an electric toothbrush in the bedroom if it is one that lights up whilst charging, or place it somewhere where the red light can't be seen.

The right mattress

We spend about a third of our lives in bed, so it is essential to have a good, supportive mattress, especially when you are experiencing discomfort. For a mattress to be fully supportive, it is recommended that it is changed every eight years. This depends on whether there are two of you sleeping on it, and/or if you are light or heavy. A well-worn mattress can give you extra aches and pains so if you wake up in the morning with back pain, it's time to think about a new one.

What you replace it with is completely subjective. Some people swear by memory foam, others don't like it. There are now hybrid mattresses which are combinations of memory foam and springs, which could provide the best of both worlds.

Be warm and cosy

If you're cold at night you are far less likely to sleep well. If you can have the heating on and controlled by a thermostat it should warm up the bedroom when it gets very cold. Having a hot water bottle or a wheatgerm bag that you heat up (which is a bit safer than a hot water bottle) means that you start off the night feeling warm. Ensure that the bedding is warm enough and wear sufficient night clothes to keep you warm in bed, including socks if necessary.

Conversely, being hot at night is very likely to wake you up. Consider fewer covers – perhaps invest in a summer duvet that is lighter, wear less in bed or on hot days keep windows open. Sleeping with just a sheet as a covering is a good option when the weather is really warm.

Be comfortable

We all have our own way of sleeping but if we are in a position that causes strain on the body, some of the benefit of sleep is lost. Having too many pillows is likely to mean that your neck is in an awkward position, raised above the body. You might have to experiment to get it right and you can start by sleeping with one pillow to see if it improves your comfort. Sleeping on either side or back is preferable to lying on your front, which can cause a painful neck.

Often people find their fingers turn inwards and they wake up with their hands in a fist, which is not good for arthritic fingers. Make a conscious effort to straighten your fingers while awake and even put your hands together (in a prayer position) to keep them flat.

Naps and exercise in the day

For some it is essential to have an afternoon nap, but this could have a detrimental effect on night-time sleep. However, if getting a good night's sleep seems impossible, it is necessary to catch up during the day.

Exercise during the day helps with sleep at night, but exercise in the evening is thought not to be helpful as it can be over-stimulating and make it more difficult to get to sleep!

On the Sleep Council's website there is a questionnaire to fill in about your sleep patterns and problems, which provides you with a '30-Day better sleep plan'. It's well worth doing – see Further information on page 128 for details.

Relaxation techniques help sleep

Quietening the mind for 10 to 20 minutes once or twice a day can be very calming, which helps with getting a better night's sleep naturally. Some older people are put off by the term 'meditation' but it simply means having some time and space where you let go of all the thoughts, worries and ideas that are buzzing through your mind.

Either lie down on your back or sit comfortably with your feet flat on the floor. Close your eyes and try to think about letting go of tension in your body and your mind. You need to be in a position that enables you to breathe freely and deeply into your diaphragm. Breathing is an important part of relaxation – breathing deeply as opposed to the shallow breathing that many of us do all the time.

Donna Farhi writes, 'Full body breathing is an extraordinary symphony of both powerful and subtle movements that massage our internal organs, oscillate our joints, and alternately tone and release all the muscles in the body. It is a full participation with life'.[1]

It often seems hard to switch off from the 'chattering mind'; that is completely normal. We go over and over the things we need to do, what someone said, how much work we have to do, and important and trivial worries. This is perfectly normal so just gently try to bring your mind back to focus on the relaxation.

How to focus the mind

- **Guided meditation**: a CD, podcast or app talks you into the relaxation, and may include visualisation, such as imagining going to one of your favourite places – a beach, garden, or somewhere in the countryside – relaxing with the warm sun on your body.

- **Counting your breath**: breathe in deeply to your diaphragm to the count of four and breathe out to four, then increase this to six if you find that possible. The benefits of breathing deeply include lowering blood pressure, improving blood flow and circulation, and calming the mind and body.
- **Transcendental meditation** (or TM) uses a mantra, which is usually a Sanskrit word that doesn't mean anything to you, and you repeat it continually while your eyes are closed. This is widely practised in India and other Asian countries. Without a mantra, you could just repeat 'one-two' to achieve a similar effect.
- **Positive affirmation** involves repeating specific words, either provided by a yoga teacher or from a book, or of your choice (as long as they are positive). For instance, you could keep repeating: 'May I be happy and healthy' and you can use any other words you like. This has a relaxing effect, like a mantra.
- **Relaxing each body part:** You can find CDs or apps which guide you, or talk yourself through tensing and relaxing every part of your body, from your feet up to your head.
- **Music**: Simply lie down and breathe deeply while emptying your mind and listen to soothing music or sounds like birdsong or other sounds of nature – waterfalls, rain, etc.

There are numerous meditations available online, on CDs and apps, many of which are free – see Further information page 128. There will be plenty of mindfulness courses available locally (see Chapter 11) which have the overall effect of helping you to relax and feel in control. Mindfulness includes a meditation element. See Further information, pages 127-128, for free online courses.

Coping with inclement weather

Old people often say they can tell what the weather is going to do because they can feel it in their joints. So it is that millions of people become amateur forecasters seemingly due to the change in barometric pressure in the atmosphere, which appears to affect our joints. Conversely, warm sunny days tend to make people feel better in themselves, but often banish aches and pains as well.

Is there any scientific evidence for this phenomenon? It may be that some people are more weather sensitive than others, as was found in research conducted in six European countries.[2] Although British people would claim that a long hot summer (as in 2018) means that they experience much less pain and inflammation, scientists have found that when people live in warm or hot climates, they still develop osteoarthritis but are less likely to suffer pain.

When the weather is warm, it is accompanied by high pressure in the atmosphere and when it is damp, rainy and cloudy the pressure is usually low, which appears to present more problems. While humidity can be a problem too, it is far more likely that damp, cold weather will give rise to aches and pains, as opposed to humid hot weather.

It may actually be the lowering of barometric pressure that affects people the most – not the pressure itself. Scientists carried out a study at Tufts University, Boston, of 200 people of around 60 years old with osteoarthritis of the knee over a three-month period.[3] They concluded that changes in barometric pressure and ambient temperature are independently associated with osteoarthritis knee pain severity. Every 10 degree drop in temperature was also linked to an increase in arthritis pain.

Similar research into 810 participants of 65 to 85 years with osteoarthritis in the hip, hands or knee was carried out in six European countries over 12 to 18 months.[4] Scientists found that there was a significant interaction effect between daily average humidity and temperature on joint pain, with the effect of humidity on pain being stronger in relatively cold weather conditions. Changes in weather variables between two consecutive days were not significantly associated with reported joint pain.

While there is some research that proves that it's not just an old wives' tale, what medical experts are not yet sure about is why a drop in temperature or changes in barometric pressure actually cause more pain. Theories put forward are that changes in barometric pressure can cause expansion or contraction of muscles, bones and tendons, causing pain, and that low temperatures might increase the consistency of joint fluids, which results in stiffness. There is no doubt that good, sunny weather makes people feel better and that dull, wet, or cold weather makes people feel more miserable – and they may focus more on their pain (see Chapter 11).

Find some winter sun (if you can)

Obviously, we can't do anything about the weather. Getting out of the winter chill and into some sunshine depends on your budget. Some people are lucky enough to be able to take a month or more as a holiday in southern Europe or in other warmer climes in winter to escape the cold, and it certainly helps them.

However, this is not likely to be realistic for many people, so we can only ensure that we stay warm in winter and take measures to make ourselves comfortable (see Chapter 9).

Wear plenty of layers

Practically speaking you can buy thermal underwear – many outlets sell a range of thermal vests with long sleeves and thermal leggings too, which are designed with fashion in mind! They are quite inexpensive to buy and ensure that your body retains warmth when the weather gets too cold. Always wrap up well when going outside with plenty of layers, from a thermal vest to a thick coat, scarf, hat, gloves and warm boots. Although we can't change the weather, we can certainly proof ourselves against it, and the more active we are the more we stay warm.

Warming the body

What else can be done? There are many ways of applying warmth and relieving pain.

- Take a hot bath with a handful of Epsom salts in the water. They are actually magnesium sulphate and have a reputation for easing aches and pains, soothing a tired body, relaxing the muscles and clearing toxins.
- A simple and easy solution is to use hot water bottles (or wheat bags are even safer, as I have said, and can be warmed in a microwave or low-heat oven).
- Add essential oils to the bath – rosemary, lavender, geranium are all soothing. Just a few drops in a bath full of water can be dispersed with your hand.
- If you're lucky enough to have access to a hot tub or jacuzzi it can be very soothing to aching joints.
- Similarly, if you can get into a sauna regularly, it's a great way of heating the body through without being in the sun.
- Whenever you wash your hands in the winter, wait for the water to get hot. Arthritic hands don't want to be immersed in cold water.
- Hot wax units are also very soothing and available in chemists. Heating up the device makes the wax melt (this requires preparation in advance). When you've turned it off test the temperature with a finger and then dip the whole hand in. The wax clings to your hand and solidifies on it keeping it very warm. (Be careful when doing this that the hot wax isn't knocked over or that you don't burn yourself when it's too hot.)

Devices to ease pain and discomfort

- **Hand-held laser**: You can invest in a small laser device which you can find online and apply to painful or swollen joints. It has a gentle warming effect. For a much stronger laser treatment you can pay privately (this is not yet available on the NHS). See Further information, page 138.
- **A TENS machine** provides a degree of pain relief through electronic currents applied through a pad placed on the affected area. TENS stands for transcutaneous electrical nerve stimulation and is widely used for pain relief in childbirth.
- **Scenar therapy** is an advanced form of non-invasive electrotherapy which uses hi-tech, computer-modulated, electrical impulses similar to those produced by your own nervous system. It is also possible to have scenar therapy from a therapist, and it is used for patients at the Margaret Hills Clinic (see Chapter 6, page 64).

Chapter 11

Lonely, depressed and stressed

This book is all about the positive things you can do to prevent osteoarthritis from becoming limiting and taking over your life. The reality is that for some people their lives have already been changed by osteoarthritis and their quality of life is seriously diminished. Surveys from the charity, Versus Arthritis (formerly Arthritis Care), highlight the emotional effect of immobility due to arthritis for a large number of people in the UK.

It's easy to see why anyone with pain, discomfort and limited mobility would find it hard to stay cheerful. Worry about the future and how to cope alone or retain independence can make people anxious. The future can seem very bleak, particularly when there seems to be no way of improving it. Depression can also result from feelings of hopelessness about the future and from a radical change in lifestyle and no longer being active. Sometimes people have to give up much-loved hobbies and activities and are unable to visit family and friends, so they feel cut off and forgotten.

Anyone who has ever felt lonely will know that it's very hard to pick yourself up and go and meet new people. Loneliness breeds lack of confidence and the longer it goes on, the less likely you are to take up a new hobby or get involved in a social activity. You may need someone to help and encourage you.

There were over 1.4 million over 50s in the UK who were

lonely in 2016/17 according to a report by Age UK, and the number is growing.[1] Loneliness is claimed to be as damaging to health as smoking 15 cigarettes a day.[2] The need to socialise and see people (or at least speak to someone) has a huge effect on health, and there are many charities and other groups that offer opportunities for people to meet others on a regular basis.

The effect of osteoarthritis

Osteoarthritis may prevent you from going out or socialising – it's quite common to feel a lack of confidence about tackling public transport, stairs or walking in busy streets. Having a social life, enjoying a much-loved activity, and/or going out usually acts as a great distraction from pain and discomfort. So, it becomes a vicious circle – staying in and not seeing people naturally leads to focusing more on health issues.

Not going out means:

- loss of independence
- lack of confidence
- inability to do things that are enjoyable
- not getting any exercise.

This can add up to feelings of despair and depression, which may eventually lead to mental illness.

Survey on mental wellbeing

Arthritis Care ran a survey in 2017 examining the impact of arthritis on mental wellbeing.[3] The survey was based on 3000 responses in the UK from people who had all types of arthritis, not just osteoarthritis, which is usually less severe. The survey found that:

- 79 per cent claimed that their condition made them feel anxious or depressed

- 50 per cent said their arthritis caused them to feel isolated or lonely
- 47 per cent admitted that their arthritis had caused them to lose contact with friends
- 80 per cent had given up hobbies or activities they enjoyed because of their health condition
- over half (54 per cent) of respondents claimed that their arthritis made it difficult to use public transport
- severe pain increased feelings of anxiety by 34 per cent, and depression by 41 per cent, compared with those who had moderate or no pain
- feelings of depression and anxiety were much more common in people who did not feel able to manage their arthritis well
- 89 per cent of respondents were worried about how arthritis would affect their future independence.

What doctors can do

There is a move towards social prescribing within the NHS, which means that doctors recognise the knock-on effect of health conditions and how important it is to look at the whole person, and not just the illness. This approach is currently being encouraged and is spreading throughout GP surgeries in the UK. Doctors aim to find out more about the whole person in front of them, asking them, 'What matters to you?' rather than, 'What is the matter with you?'

So far, not everyone has access to doctors who take this approach, but it is a growing movement. Dr Michael Dixon, Chair of the College of Medicine and Integrated Health, NHS England National Clinical Champion Lead for Social Prescription, and a GP in Devon, reports that in Rotherham, Yorkshire, where this approach has been adopted for those that use hospital services most, there has been a 20 per cent reduction in GP consultations and hospital admissions and that after three years the over-80s are using hospitals up to 50 per cent less.

Improving your quality of life

It is hard for people who feel isolated to pick themselves up and join a group, particularly if they are worried about how they are going to get there. When a doctor facilitates this for them, it can make it feel more accessible and easier.

Activities which can help change your mood

There are all kinds of mood-boosting activities that can be accessible, such as tai chi or yoga, gardening, cooking, sewing, playing bridge or other card games, pottery, learning English, or joining a reading group. Activity is mentally cheering as well as doing you good physically. The social element of being in a group of people on a regular basis is uplifting and is usually relatively inexpensive.

Other things you can do too which may make you feel happy include:

- **Singing**: There's nothing like opening up and singing even if you were told as a young person that you didn't have a singing voice. Check out local choirs, or singing groups, including sound and music healing.
- **Music**: Listening to music can transport you to another world. Make sure you have the facility to listen to your favourite music, whatever it is.
- **Radio and podcasts**: There are so many stations now, particularly on digital, make sure you have a good radio, tablet or other device to find the programmes you enjoy.
- **Walking**: Joining a local group means that you meet people, get out in nature, and have much-needed exercise as well.
- **Pets**: If it's practical, how about getting a cat or dog? Pets

can give company and comfort and make you feel less alone.

All over the country local groups are run by charities such as Versus Arthritis (formerly Arthritis Care) and Arthritis Action. The local support groups or arthritis action groups enable people to get together regularly with those who are in the same situation. These groups have interesting speakers, including health professionals, organise sessions with complementary therapists, and arrange fundraising events. At a meeting everyone is encouraged to discuss what works for them and as a group they can have greater influence and find out more about local services – which may include day care centres.

The charity, Contact the Elderly, holds free Sunday afternoon tea parties once a month, and volunteers offer lifts to the venue.

See Further information on pages 125 to find out more about help and groups.

What you can do at home

Recent figures from Age UK[1] found that 2 million people over 75 live alone. A million of these claim that they can go for a month without speaking to a friend, family member or neighbour. It takes courage to change this situation and sometimes someone else needs to do it for you.

If going out proves impossible, it helps to speak to someone regularly on the phone. Age UK offers a weekly friendship call on the phone for those who don't have any friends or family to speak to.

Modern technology enables you to speak to people all over the world for free for as long as you like. So, if you have family or friends who you don't see very often but who you would like to chat to regularly it's possible to do this with a computer, tablet or smart phone through many different services (such as FaceTime, Viber and Skype). Although this can sound daunting to some people, it is easy to do and enables personal contact and the chance to see the grandchildren on the screen and chat to them. Age UK provides information about how to do this.

Getting emotional support

Mental wellbeing is as important as physical health, but it is believed by many that there is a strong connection between mind and body, and it is widely accepted that stress can both cause illness and make it worse. Complementary therapists believe that our emotions can cause disease through the tension and pressure that we put on certain parts of our body.

Just think about how you feel when you are nervous – butterflies, upset stomach; imagine feeling like that all the time. Similarly, when we are depressed or feeling overburdened, we tend to raise and/or hunch our shoulders, and eventually muscles become fixed and painful and we develop a permanent stoop.

If you feel like this, your first port of call should be your GP where you can explain how you feel. Doctors vary in their approach and some are likely to prescribe antidepressants, which may be appropriate if you have suffered recent trauma or bereavement as they can get you through a very bad phase.

People need hope, and ageing combined with arthritis can be a worrying time. Learning to feel more relaxed through meditation, mindfulness and autogenic training, can make you feel stronger and happier. Autogenic training encourages people to access their own physical relaxation process and use it to relieve physical and emotional stress. It originates from research on hypnosis, and has been compared to yoga and meditation, which influence the body's autonomic nervous system (see Further information).

However, if you are lonely and depressed in general, perhaps partly due to your arthritis, it is often helpful to be referred to someone to talk to who is not emotionally involved with you.

Talking therapies

Addressing emotional issues through talking therapies may also help with pain management in addition to some of the practical and physical suggestions mentioned in previous chapters. It can also help to discover different approaches to ease pain and discomfort.

There are various ways of getting counselling and other talking therapies which are sometimes free, but quite often have to be paid for. If you are in the UK, access to talking therapies on the NHS can take a long time depending on where you live. Check with your doctor what availability there is in your area. The therapy provided by the NHS is usually CBT (cognitive behavioural therapy, see next page) rather than counselling.

Counselling

Seeing a counsellor is about having time just for you to express exactly what you feel, in confidence, without being judged and with a person who is emotionally objective, unlike family members and friends.

Discussing current and past problems with a trained counsellor or psychotherapist and discovering your own patterns of behaviour can help to make the difference between serious depression, loneliness and anxiety and feeling more positive about life. Some people hold on to past hurts and traumas all their lives without talking about them and find that being with a counsellor provides the opportunity to air these problems and start to let them go.

Counselling can help with any form of mental stress or illness, anxiety, depression, grief or despair. It can also have a knock-on effect on physical symptoms because stress adversely affects our bodies.

Most counsellors are private, but some churches and other organisations provide access to therapy at a reduced price. You can enquire at the doctor's or contact Versus Arthritis. See Further information on page 124 for how to find a local counsellor.

CBT (cognitive behavioural therapy)

Cognitive behavioural therapy looks at changing behaviour by examining unwanted and negative beliefs and thoughts. Although it is understood that these negative thoughts and behaviour patterns have their roots in the past, CBT does not delve deeply into early life.

It is quite common for humans not to understand their own behaviour or where their feelings come from. CBT therapists use structured techniques to identify the thinking behind negative feelings and behaviour and teach skills to allow people to make changes and respond to events more positively.

To find out about NHS or online CBT courses go to Further information, pages 126-127.

Meditation and mindfulness

There is plenty of mystique around meditation but there is no need for there to be. As explained in earlier chapters, by sitting quietly, closing your eyes, concentrating on breathing and repeating a word or counting to yourself for around 20 minutes you usually find that you feel much calmer. If you do have this quiet time every day, after a few weeks there is a greater sense of relaxation and of being able to cope with health and other problems better.

Alternatively, you can find a local meditation group, which can make it easier to be disciplined and focus. Check online, or in newsagents' windows, local papers, or at the library or doctor's surgery.

Mindfulness means being aware of yourself – your feelings and actions – and also comprises meditation. There are four main principals of mindfulness:

- letting go – not holding on to past grievances and hurts
- acceptance – realising that some things just are, and that you cannot do anything to change them
- presence – in line with the Buddhist concept of living in the now, instead of dwelling on the past and imagining the future (which rarely turns out to be as we expect it to be)
- perception – being aware of what is going on around you and specifically with yourself and your feelings.

Whatever these principles sound like to you, they usually take some time to become natural, so no-one can expect to integrate them immediately. To help with developing a calmer mind and body and focusing clearly, mindfulness always includes meditation. The benefits of meditation make it easier to be aware of when there is a need to concentrate on these four tenets to help yourself and those around you, and to cope with difficult situations.

By being more conscious of your thoughts and feelings you become more able to cope with them and make considered decisions. Both mindfulness and meditation can enable you to stop focusing on pain and get some welcome respite, and they are now employed widely in pain management. The aim is to accept the pain and alleviate the emotional reaction attached to it. This involves acknowledging that pain is there, but detaching yourself from it removes the power that it had over your mind before, making it easier to bear.

Mindfulness is being used in the NHS for pain management. UCLH (University College London Hospital) has a helpful audio guide entitled, *Self-help resources for pain management* (see Further information, page 128).

Natural alternatives to antidepressants

As outlined in earlier chapters, herbal remedies can make you feel less tense and upset without any side-effects – see Chapter 7.

Yoga uses breathing techniques and postures that are designed to boost physical and mental wellbeing and therefore can be good for depression and stress. Tai chi is a calming, meditative form of exercise that encourages wellbeing and relaxation – see Chapter 4.

Many of the complementary therapies outlined in Chapter 8 are both relaxing and stress relieving. Many are therapeutic because of the attention and pampering element, of having someone who listens to you and aims to make you feel good.

Chapter 12

Soups, juices and meals with turmeric and ginger

Turmeric is one of the new 'superfoods'. For many of us who have been using this deep yellow spice for curries for the last 40 years, it's surprising to see the turmeric latte, golden milks, and turmeric tea available in well-known coffee shops. That's all testament to the many health properties that this humble spice has had attributed to its name.

As I said in Chapter 7 (page 68), it is the *curcumin* in turmeric that is the essential ingredient. This is extracted using alcohol or cooking in oil with the addition of black pepper, which enhances the absorption of curcumin. There is plenty of research about turmeric,[2] and you can read more about turmeric supplements and the benefits of it in Chapter 7; for supplement suppliers, look in Further information, page 135.

Ginger hasn't ever received the acclaim it deserves and for many years its use was considered simply for sweet recipes, to make crystallised ginger or gingerbread men and in fizzy drinks – ginger beer and ginger ale. More recently it has also become trendy like turmeric and is often found in freshly made and bottled juices. It is also a key component of spicy meals and is often drunk as a tea.

The active ingredient in ginger is *gingerol,* which has powerful anti-inflammatory properties, so, if it is to your taste, it's well worth drinking and cooking with ginger. It is also a warming herb and said to improve the circulation. In Ayurvedic medicine (from the Indian subcontinent) it is eaten widely in winter; the principle is to relate the appropriate type of food eaten to the season.

Turmeric recipes

Be aware that turmeric is used as a natural dye and will end up colouring your kitchen surfaces and clothes bright yellow if you're not careful with it. It will make your hands yellow too!

Turmeric paste is very popular and is helpful in easing the pain and inflammation of arthritis in people, and in dogs. It involves heating up turmeric powder in water, and then adding coconut oil and black pepper, a vital ingredient to help absorption in the body. After making up the paste, keep a jar in the fridge and add a teaspoonful to meals. Make sure it is mixed in properly or it can result in a rather strong coughing reaction! The action of heating the coconut oil extracts the curcumin, and adding the black pepper containing *piperine* enhances the bioavailability of curcumin.

Golden turmeric smoothie
(Dr Susan Aldridge, medical blogger)

The anti-inflammatory properties of turmeric are well known and the subject of over 6000 scientific papers demonstrating its potential power against cancer, diabetes, arthritis and a range of other conditions. So here is a blender berry smoothie with added turmeric, which turns the drink into a lovely peach-gold colour. Fresh cranberries are included here, which can be juiced when they are in season but, for a sweeter drink, substitute blueberries, raspberries, strawberries or a mixture.

Serves one

½ tsp turmeric powder
250 ml (8 fl oz) hemp or almond milk
1 banana
2.5 cm/1 inch peeled and chopped ginger root
100 g (4 oz) fresh cranberries
1 tsp cacao powder

- Blast all the ingredients in the blender and drink immediately.

Yellow split pea dahl

(Dr Susan Aldridge, medical blogger)

Serves four

  2 onions
  3 cloves garlic
  Spices: include a mixture of black mustard seeds, fennel seeds and
      cumin seeds, all blasted in a grinder or ground in a pestle and
      mortar, plus one teaspoon each of ground turmeric and ground
      cinnamon.
  2 tbsp tomato purée
  1 tbsp chilli jam
  100 g (4 oz) red lentils
  100 g (4 oz) yellow split peas
  400 ml (14 fl oz) water
  1 bag frozen peas or mixed veg

- Fry the onion and garlic in coconut oil, then add the spices, tomato purée and chilli jam. Cook for around 10 minutes, until soft.
- Then stir in the lentils and split peas and add the water.
- Cook until soft and then add the mixed vegetables, cooking for a few more minutes.

This is a good dish to serve over two days. Day one, add a baked sweet potato and the next day, re-heat and serve with 200 g (7 oz) basmati rice (or similar) with some interesting additions (I used one with pinto beans, chilli and lime – there are lots of options). A dollop of mint and cucumber raita and some mango chutney wouldn't go amiss either.

Turmeric rainbow juice
(Dr Susan Aldridge, medical blogger)

Serves one

3 oranges, peeled and halved
3 carrots, peeled and roughly chopped
1 small beetroot, roughly chopped
handful kale (or spinach)
5 cm/2 inches turmeric root, peeled
5 cm/2 inches ginger root, peeled

- Juice everything and drink immediately.

Ginger and turmeric recipes

Moroccan spiced cauliflower soup

(from *Easy. Tasty. Healthy.* by Barbara Cousins)

Serves two to four

- ½ cauliflower (about 400 g/14 oz) broken into florets and stem sliced
- 1 onion, diced
- 2.5 cm (1inch) piece of fresh root ginger, peeled and grated
- 1 stock cube dissolved in 1.2 litres (2 pints) boiling water
- 1 tsp ground cinnamon
- 1 tsp ground cumin
- ½ tsp garam masala
- ½ tsp turmeric
- seeds from 10 cardamom pods, crushed
- 50 g (2 oz) ground almonds
- salt and lots of freshly ground black pepper
- paprika for sprinkling

- Place the vegetables, ginger, stock and spices in a saucepan and bring to the boil.
- Reduce the heat and simmer for 5–8 minutes or until the vegetables are just cooked.
- Add the ground almonds and blend the soup until smooth.
- Season to taste with salt and pepper and add a sprinkling of paprika to serve.

Indian chicken curry

(Frances Ive)

Serves four

4 chicken breasts

250 g (9 oz) plain yoghurt (cow's, goat's, soy or coconut)

3 onions

3 cloves garlic

2.5 cm/1 inch piece of fresh root ginger (or 1 tbsp ground ginger)

1–2 tsp chilli

1 tsp ground turmeric

1 tsp ground coriander

1 tsp ground cumin

pinch Himalayan crystal salt (or unrefined sea salt)

1 tsp ground cloves

⅛ packet creamed coconut

½ tsp mustard

2 tbsp ghee (or coconut oil)

1 tsp cinnamon

1 lemon, juiced

coriander leaves

- Marinate the chicken pieces in yoghurt and salt for 6 hours.
- Slice the onions, garlic and ginger, and brown them lightly in oil.
- Add all the remaining ingredients except for the coriander leaves and lemon juice. Fry for a few minutes, stirring to prevent burning.
- Add the chicken in its marinade and cook on a brisk heat, stirring until the meat is reddish brown and dry.
- Add 2 cups of hot water and simmer, covered, on a low heat until the chicken is tender.
- When the chicken is nearly cooked, add the coriander.

Cauliflower curry

(Frances Ive)

Serves two to four

    2.5 cm (1 inch) piece of fresh root ginger

    2 garlic cloves

    2 red onions

    1 large cauliflower

    1 dsp coconut oil

    1 tsp ground turmeric

    1 tsp ground cumin

    1 tsp ground coriander

    1 tsp cumin seeds

    Approx. ½ a 500 g (8 oz) carton of plain yoghurt (soy, coconut, cow's or goat's)

    creamed coconut (1 sachet or ¼ of a block) or 400 ml tin (14 fl oz) coconut milk

- Fry the ginger root, garlic and onions for a few minutes in the coconut oil, then add all the spices.
- Cut up the cauliflower into bite-sized pieces and add to the pan.
- Fry on a low heat for 10 minutes (checking that there is enough coconut oil).
- Add the yoghurt and coconut, stir well and cook gently until the cauliflower is soft and ready to eat.
- Serve with brown basmati rice.

Further information

Help and advice for osteoarthritis and older people

Versus Arthritis: UK charity, the former Arthritis Care and Arthritis Research combined, offers services and support for people with arthritis. Branches and groups all over the country meet regularly for talks and outings.

Helpline: 0808 800 4050
Website: www.versusarthritis.org

Arthritis Action: A charity that helps people to manage their arthritis, offering help and advice on weight loss, healthy eating, exercise, and runs local groups.

Freephone: 0800 652 3188
Website: www.arthritisaction.org.uk

The Arthritis Foundation: US charity providing information and services. Publishes *Arthritis Today*.

Website: www.arthritis.org

Arthritis Ireland
Website: www.arthritisireland.ie

Contact the Elderly: Runs tea parties for the over 75s one Sunday a month.
> Freephone: 0800 716543
> Website: www.contact-the-elderly.org.uk

Independent Age: Gives advice and help to elderly people.
> Freephone: 0800 319 6789
> Email: advice@independentage.org
> Website: www.independentage.org

Independent Living: news, advice and products relating to improving life with disability
> Website: www.independentliving.co.uk/about/

The Disabled Living Foundation: Has a very helpful website, AskSara, which does an online assessment and suggests products that can make living at home much easier, as well as indicating how to get these free of charge if eligible.
> Website: asksara.dlf.org.uk

The Silver Line: A helpline for older people set up by Esther Rantzen.
> Freephone: 08004 708090
> Website: www.silverage.org.uk

Age UK: Helpline, voluntary help, and local groups around the country.
> Freephone: 0800 055 6112
> Website: www.ageuk.org.uk

Age Action Ireland
> Website: www.ageaction.ie

Friends of the Elderly: Offer a weekly or fortnightly friendship call from a volunteer who enjoys talking to older people.
> Phone: 0300 332 1110
> Website: www.fote.org.uk/

Friends of the Elderly, Ireland
Website: https://friendsoftheelderly.ie/

National Health Service, UK (NHS)
Website: www.nhs.uk

NHS: information on preventing falls.
Website: www.nhs.uk/conditions/falls/prevention

Country Living: Magazine running a campaign that matches older people with dogs.
Website: www.countryliving.com/uk/wildlife/pets/
a20770696/

Pedigree Food: Dog food manufacturer also with campaign matching older people with dogs.
Website: uk.pedigree.com/dogdates

British Geriatrics Society: Improving healthcare for older people.
Website: www.bgs.org.uk

Emotional support

Talking therapies

Association of Professional Counsellors & Psychotherapists in Ireland (APCP)
Website: www.apcp.ie/find-a-counsellor-psychotherapist/

British Association for Counselling and Psychotherapy
Phone: 01455 883300
Twitter: @bacp
Website: www.bacp.co.uk

British Association of Behavioural and Cognitive Psychotherapies
Phone: 01254 875277
Website: www.babcp.com

CBT treatment on the NHS: You can refer yourself.
Website: beta.nhs.uk/find-a-psychological-therapies-service

Irish Council for Psychotherapy
Website: www.psychotherapycouncil.ie/find/

Irish Association for Counselling & Psychotherapy (IACP)
Website: https://iacp.ie

Irish Association of Humanistic and Integrative
 Psychotherapy (IAHIP)
Website: https://iahip.org/

Irish Council for Psychotherapy (ICP)
Website: www.psychotherapycouncil.ie/

The Westminster Pastoral Foundation
Phone: 020 7361 4800
Website: www.wpf.org.uk

Cruse Bereavement Care Helpline
Phone: 0870 167 1677
Young person's helpline: 0808 808 1677
Website: www.crusebereavementcare.org.uk

Relate: For relationship advice.
Phone: 0207 456 1310
Website: www.relate.org.uk

Mindfulness

Future Learn: (part of the Open University) runs mindfulness
courses online which are completely free of charge.
Website: www.futurelearn.com/courses

UCLH (University College of London Hospital) offers an online eight-week course in mindfulness and provides several mindfulness meditations aimed at pain management entitled: *Self-help resources for pain management.*
Website: www.uclh.nhs.uk

Be Mindful Online
Website: www.bemindfulonline.com

Insight Timer
Website: www.insighttimer.com

Headspace
Website: www.headspace.co.uk

Sleep

The Sleep Council: Fill in the 30 Day Better Sleep Plan questionnaire for guidance on how to sleep better.
Website: https://sleepcouncil.org.uk

Practitioners and associations

Acupuncture

British Acupuncture Council
Phone: 020 8735 0400
Webiste: www.acupuncture.org.uk

Acupuncture Council of Ireland
Website: www.acupuncturecouncilofireland.com/
find-an-acupuncturist

Alison Savory, BSc (Hons), DipTN, LicAc, MBAcC, PhD
Acupuncture and East Asian Medicine Health Practitioner, Barnstaple, Devon.
Email: alison@oneacupuncture.co.uk
Website: www.oneacupuncture.co.uk

Alexander Technique

Society of Teachers of the Alexander Technique (STAT)
Phone: 0208 885 6524
Website: www.stat.org.uk

Ian O'Donnell, Alexander Technique practitioner, Surrey.
Email: ianodonnell@btinternet.com
Phone: 07909 796168

ITM (Interactive Teaching Method)
Website: itmalexandertechnique.org
www.alexandertechnique-itm.ie

Alexander Technique in Ireland
Website: www.alexander.ie/findateacher.html

Aromatherapy

The Aromatherapy Council
Website: www.aromatherapycouncil.org.uk
www.ptcny.net/clients/ARC/RA/Public/Search.aspx

Ayurveda

Anandaspa, India.
Website: www.anandaspa.com

Bowen Therapy

BTPA
Phone: 017713 552858
Website: www.bowentherapy.org.uk

College of Bowen Studies
Website: https://thebowentechnique.com/practitioners/
find-a-practitioner/

Chiropractic

General Chiropractic Council
    Phone: 020 7713 5155
    Website: www.gcc-uk.org

British Chiropractic Association
    Phone: 01506 639 607
    Website: www.chiropractic-uk.co.uk

McTimoney Chiropractic Association
    Phone: 01491 739120
    Website: www.mctimoney-chiropractic.org

Cider vinegar

The Margaret Hills Clinic, Warwickshire, specialises in treatments with cider vinegar.
    Phone: 01926 854783
    Website: www.margarethillsclinic.com

Emmett Technique

    Emmett UK (for the UK and Ireland)
    Website: https://emmett-uk.com/contact

Homeopathy

British Homeopathic Association
    Phone: 0203 640 5903
    Website: www.trusthomeopathy.org

The Society of Homeopaths
    Phone: 01604 817890
    Website: https://homeopathy-soh.org/

Irish Society of Homeopaths
> Website: https://irishhomeopathy.ie/list/find_
> homeopaths/

Ann-Louise Holland
> Phone: 07770841840
> Email: Ann-louise@kanshabrands.com

Herbal medicine

The National Institute of Medical Herbalists
> Phone: 01392 426022
> Website: www.nimh.org.uk

Register of Chinese Herbal Medicine
> Phone: 01603 927420
> Website: www.rchm.co.uk

Ayurvedic Professional Association
> Phone: 01273 257077
> Website: apa.uk.com/find-a-practitioner

Irish Register of Herbalists
> Website: https://irh.ie/find-an-irh-registered-herbalist-in-
> your-area/

Dr Christopher J. Etheridge PhD MRSC,MCPP CChem DoIC
ARCS BSc (Hons) Chem BSc (Hons) Phyto,
Medical herbalist, Central London & Epping.
> Phone: 0777 941 4099
> Website: www.chrisetheridgeherbalist.co.uk

Naturopathy

Complementary & Natural Healthcare Council
> Website: https://cnhcregister.org.uk/newsearch/

General Council and Register of Naturopaths, British Naturopathic Association
Phone: 01458 840072
Website: www.naturopathy.org.uk

Nutrition

Association of Naturopathic Practitioners - Nutritionists
Website: https://theanp.co.uk/Nutritional-Therapy

British Association for Nutrition and Lifestyle Medicine
Phone: 01425 462532
Website: www.bant.org.uk
Find a practitioner: https://bant.org.uk/bant/jsp/
practitionerSearch.faces

British Society for Ecological Medicine
Website: www.bsem.org.uk/pages/14-practitioners

Centre for Nutrition Education & Lifestyle Management
Website: https://cnelm.co.uk/clinic/find-practitioner/

Institute for Optimum Nutrition
Phone: 020 8614 7800
Website: www.ion.ac.uk

International Institute of Nutrition and Health
Website: www.iinh.net/find-a-practitioner/

Osteopathy

The General Osteopathic Council
Phone: 020 7357 6655
Website: www.osteopathy.org.uk

Osteopathic Council of Ireland
Website: www.osteopathy.ie/find-an-osteopath

Oxygen therapy

The Hyperbaric Oxygen Therapy Centre
Phone: 0203 8231212
Website: www.hyperbaricoxygentherapy.co.uk

National Hyperbaric Centre, Dublin
Website: http://hyperbaricireland.com/

Physiotherapy

Sammy Margo, Chartered Physiotherapist, London in private practice and spokesperson for the Chartered Society of Physiotherapy.
Phone: 020 7435 4910
Website: www.sammymargophysiotherapy.com

Chartered Society of Physiotherapy
Website: www.csp.org.uk/

Irish Society of Chartered Physiotherapists
Website: www.iscp.ie/why-choose-chartered/find-chartered-physiotherapists

Pilates

Body Control Pilates Association
Phone: 0207 636 8900
Website: www.bodycontrolpilates.com

Brigitte Tetlow, Surrey.
Website: www.pilateswithbrigitte.co.uk

Lynne Robinson, founder of Body Control Pilates
Website: www.bodycontrolpilates.com

Reflexology

Association of Reflexologists
   Phone: 01823 351010
   Website: www.aor.org.uk

Irish Reflexologists Institute
   Website: www.reflexology.ie / find-a-reflexologist /

Reiki

The Reiki Association
   Website: www.reikiassociation.org.uk

Reiki Federation of Ireland
   Website: www.reikifederationireland.com / MainList.php

Rheumatologists

Dr Roger Wolman, Royal National Orthopaedic Hospital.

Dr Rod Hughes, St Peter's Hospital, Chertsey, Surrey.

Tai chi

The Tai Chi Union for Great Britain
   Website: www.taichiunion.com

Yoga

British Wheel of Yoga
   Phone: 01529 306851
   Website: www.bwy.org.uk

Richard Kravetz, London.
   Website: www.yogaforall-uk.com

Slimming clubs

Weight Watchers
Email: uk.help@weightwatchers.co.uk
Website: www.weightwatchers.co.uk

Rosemary Conley
Phone: 01509 620222
Website: www.rosemaryconley.com

Slimming World
Phone: 0344 892 0400
Website: www.slimmingworld.co.uk/

Lighter Life
Phone: 08700 664747
Website: www.lighterlife.co.uk

Supplements

Turmeric/curcumin

Pukka Wholistic Organic Turmeric (620 mg)
Viridian Organic Curcumin Latte
Viridian High Potency Curcumin Complex
Viridian Organic Curcumin Extract
Viridian Organic Turmeric 400 g

Joint health

Viridian Joint Complex (vegan glucosamine 2KCI, manganese,
   vitamin C, turmeric, *Boswellia serrata*, L-proline, quercetin,
   bromelain, ginger root)
Terranova Joint Support Complex (Boswellia resin,
   enzymatically-active, fresh freeze dried botanicals: stinging
   nettle, turmeric, ginger and celery, MSM, vitamin C,
   manganese, selenium and molybdenum)

Bone Health Complex (magnesium citrate, calcium citrate,
      vitamin C (ascorbic acid), vitamin K, malic acid, boron
      (sodium borate), vitamin D3 – vegan)
Future You Health Cool Joints – 250 g of *Boswellia serrata*
Viridian Hyaluronic Acid (vegan/vegetarian)

Magnesium

Better You Magnesium Oil Joint with glucosamine and menthol
      spray
Salus Haus Magnesium Liquid Mineral Supplement

Niacin (vitamin B3)

Patrick Holford No Blush Niacin (1000 mg),
      magnesium (290 mg) and vitamin C (490 mg)
Nature's Aid No Blush Niacin, 500 mg

Vitamin B complex

Vega Vitamin B Complex Formula 30 Vegicaps
Terranova B-Complex with Vitamin C 50 caps

Omega-3

Viridian Organic Joint Omega Oil 200 ml
Equazen Naturally Sourced Omega-3 and Omega-6
Higher Nature Omega-3 Fish Oil (1000 mg)

Vitamin C

Active Edge™ CherryActive 100% concentrated Montmorency
      cherry juice
Viridian Ester-C 950 mg

Vitamin D

Better You DLux 3000 OralVit D3 (vitamin D) Spray, 15 ml
Viridian Vitamin D3 1000 or 2000 iu

Glucosamine

Biocare Glucosamine MSM Complex (Glucosamine
hydrochloride, MSM, chondoitrin sulphate)

Rosehip

GOPO® Joint Health Rosehip/GOPO, vitamin C
Litozin Rosehip and vitamin C

Herbal remedies

A Vogel Atrogel Arnica gel
Nelson's Arnicare Arnica gel
A Vogel Atrozan® Devil's Claw tablets
A Vogel Dormeasan Valerian Hops Oral Drops, 50 ml
Bach Flowers, Rescue Remedy drops, spray, pastilles and
Rescue Night drops and spray
Tiger Balm ointment (contains camphor, menthol, cajuput oil
and clove oil)
Wood Lock, Wong To Yick, Chinese medicated analgesic oil for
joints (contains wintergreen)

Bathing

Better You Magnesium Flakes, 1 kg
Teals Epsom Salts: Relax and Relief (Eucalyptus/Spearmint);
Soothe and Sleep (Lavender); Pre and Post Workout

Books

Cousins B. *Easy, Tasty, Healthy*. Harper Thorsons. 2016.

Cousins B. *Cooking Without*. Harper Thorsons. 2012.

Cousins B. *Vegetarian Cooking Without*. Harper Thorsons. 2000.

Cousins B. *Cooking Without Made Easy*. Harper Thorsons. 2005.

Hemsley J. *East by West: Simple Recipes for Ultimate Mind-Body Balance*. Macmillan. 2018.

Hay H. *You Can Heal Your Life*. Hay House. 1984.

Williams M, Penman D. *Mindfulness, a practical guide to Finding Peace in a Frantic World*. Piatkus. 2011.

Holford P. *Say No to Arthritis*. Piatkus. 2006.

Myhill S, Robinson C. *The Infection Game: Life is an Arms Race*. Hammersmith Books. 2018.

Hills M. *Treating Arthritis the Drug Free Way*. Sheldon Press. 2012.

Feuerstein G. *Yoga Gems: A Treasury of Practical and Spiritual Wisdom from Ancient and Modern Masters*. Bantam Books. 2002.

Food blogs and recipes

Dr Susan Aldridge
Website: www.susanmaldridge.com

Campaigns

On Your Feet Britain
Website: www.onyourfeetday.com

Drinkaware
Website: www.drinkaware.co.uk

Laser treatment

K Laser, powerful laser treatment. Available for animals at veterinary surgeons throughout the UK, and for humans at selected private health clinics.
Website: www.klaser.co.uk

Scenar Therapy
www.scenartherapist.co.uk

Autogenic Training
> www.autogenic-therapy.org.uk

Products

Cider vinegar:
> Biona Organic Cider Vinegar with the Mother (from health food stores).

Herbamare Herbal Salt:
> sea salt, organically grown vegetables, garden herbs and iodine-rich kelp (from health food stores – check with a doctor if you have a thyroid problem)

Backfriend – back support for a chair from MEDesign
> Website: www.medesign.co.uk/

The Healthy Back Handbag Company
> Website: www.thehealthybackbag.co.uk

Hand-held laser device – Handy Cures

Penclic: ergonomic keyboards and computer mice.
> Website: www.penclic.se

Varidesk standing desks
> Phone: 020 3808 5398
> Website: uk.varidesk.com

Comfortable shoes

> Hotter Shoes
> Website: www.hotter.com

> Skechers
> Website: www.skechers.com

> Fit Flops
> Website: www.fitflop.com

References

Chapter 1: Good health and osteoarthritis

1. Arthritis Research UK (now Versus Arthritis). *Osteoarthritis in General Practice*. 2013. healthinnovationnetwork.com/resources/osteoarthritis-in-general-practice-arthritis-research-uk-2013/ (accessed 14 May 2019).

2. NRAS. *What is RA?* www.nras.org.uk/what-is-ra-article (accessed 18 June 2019).

3. Murray C et al. UK health performance: findings of the Global Burden of Disease Study 2010. *Lancet* 2013;381 (9871): 970-972.

4. National Joint Registry for England and Wales. *15th Annual Report*. http://www.njrcentre.org.uk/njrcentre/Reports-Publications-and-Minutes (accessed 20 May 2019).

5. Mobasheri A, Rayman MP, Gualillo O, Sellam J, van der Kraan P, Fearon U. The role of metabolism in the pathogenesis of osteoarthritis. *National Review of Rheumatology* 2017;13(5):302-311.

6. Myhill S, Robinson C. *The Infection Game: Life is an Arms Race*. London: Hammersmith Health Books; 2018.

7. dos Santos Duarte Lana JF, Rodrigues BL. Osteoarthritis as a chronic inflammatory disease: A review of the inflammatory markers. In Toumi H, Mazor M (eds) *Osteoarthritis Biomarkers and Treatments*. IntechOpen. 2019. www.intechopen.com/books/osteoarthritis-biomarkers-and-treatments (accessed 20 May 2019).

Chapter 2: Looking at weight loss

1. Arthritis Research UK (now Versus Arthritis). *The State of Musculoskeletal Health 2018*. www.arthritisresearchuk. org/arthritis-information/data-and-statistics/state-of-musculoskeletal-health.aspx (accessed 20 May 2019).

2. Anderson J, Felson D. Factors associated with osteoarthritis of the knee in the first national Health and Nutrition Examination Survey (HANES I): Evidence for an association with overweight, race, and physical demands of work. *American Journal of Epidemiology* 1998;128(1):179-189.

3. Felson D, Anderson J, Naimark A, Walker A, Meenan R. Obesity and knee osteoarthritis: The Framingham Study. *Annals of Internal Medicine* 1998; 109(1):18-24.

4. Lohmander L, Gerhardsson de Verdier M, Rollof J, Nilsson P, Engström G. Incidence of severe knee and hip osteoarthritis in relation to different measures of body mass: a population-based prospective cohort study. *Annals of the Rheumatic Diseases* 2009;(68:4): 490-496.

5. Felson DT, Zhang Y, Anthony JM, Naimark, A, Anderson, JJ. Weight loss reduces the risk for symptomatic knee osteoarthritis in women. *Annals of Internal Medicine* 1992;(116):535-539.

6. Messier SP, Gutekunst DJ, Davis C, DeVita P. Weight loss reduces knee-joint loads in overweight and obese older adults with knee osteoarthritis. *Arthritis & Rheumatism* 2005; (52)7: 2026-2032.

7. Harvard Health Publishing. Why weight matters when it comes to joint pain. *HEALTHbeat*. www.health.harvard.edu/pain/why-weight-matters-when-it-comes-to-joint-pain (accessed 20 May 2019).

Chapter 3: Finding exercises to suit you

1. Kvam S, Kleppe CL, Nordhus IH, Hovland A. Exercise as a treatment for depression: A meta-analysis. *Journal Affective Disorders* 2016;(202):67-86.

Chapter 4: Exercises to protect and strengthen your body

1. Del-Pino-Casado R, Obrero-Gaitán E, Lomas-Vega R. The effect of tai chi on reducing the risk of falling: A systematic review and meta-analysis. *American Journal of Chinese Medicine* 2016;44(5):895-906.
2. Lomas-Vega R, Obrero-Gaitán E, Molina-Ortega FJ, Del-Pino-Casado R. Reply to: Comment on tai chi for risk of falls: A meta-analysis. *Journal of American Geriatric Society* 2017;65(12):2748-2749.
3. Huang ZG, Feng YH, Li YH, Lv CS. Systematic review and meta-analysis: Tai chi for preventing falls in older adults. *BMJ Open* 2017;7(2):e013661.
4. Taylor D, Hale L, Schluter P, Waters DL, Binns EE, McCracken H, McPherson K, Wolf SL. Effectiveness of tai chi as a community-based falls prevention intervention: A randomized controlled trial. *Journal of the American Geriatrics Society* 2012; 60(5):841-848.
5. Wang C, Schmid CH, Iversen MD, Harvey WF, Fielding RA, Driban JB, Price LL, Wong JB, Reid KF, Rones R, McAlindon T. Comparative effectiveness of tai chi versus physical therapy for knee osteoarthritis: A randomized trial. *Annals Internal Medicine* 2016; 165(2): 77–86.
6. Jahnke R, Larkey L, Rogers C, Etnier J, Lin F. A comprehensive review of health benefits of qigong and tai chi. *American Journal Health Promotion* 2010;24(6):e1-e25.

Chapter 5: What is healthy eating?

1. Foreman KJ, Marquez N, Dolgert A, Fukutaki K, Fullman N, McGaughey M, et al. Forecasting life expectancy, years of life lost, and all-cause and cause-specific mortality for 250 causes of death: reference and alternative scenarios for 2016–40 for 195 countries and territories. *The Lancet* 2018; 392(10159):2052-90.
2. Dyer J, Davison G, Marcora SM, Mauger AR. Effect of a Mediterranean type diet on inflammatory and cartilage degradation biomarkers in patients with osteoarthritis. *Journal of Nutritional Health Aging* 2017;21(5):562-566.
3. Han HS, Chang CB, Lee DC, Lee JY. Relationship between total

fruit and vegetable intake and self-reported knee pain in older adults. *Journal of Nutritional Health Aging* 2017;21(7):750-758.

4. Loef M, Schoones JW, Kloppenburg M, Ioan-Facsinay A. Fatty acids and osteoarthritis: different types, different effects. *Joint Bone Spine* 2018;(18):30182-9.

5. National Statistics. *Statistics on Alcohol: England, 2017* NHS Digital. 3 May 2017. https://webarchive.nationalarchives.gov.uk/20180328130416/and http://digital.nhs.uk/catalogue/PUB23940 (accessed 24 June 2019).

6. Meneton P, Jeunemaitre X, de Wardener HE, MacGregor GA. Links between dietary salt intake, renal salt handling, blood pressure, and cardiovascular diseases. *Physiology Review* 2005;85(2):679-715.

7. BBC News. What's the evidence for the gluten-free lifestyle? *BBC News*, 8 September 2016. www.bbc.co.uk/news/magazine-37292174 (accessed 24 June 2019).

Chapter 7: Supplements and herbs

1. Heisel J, Kipshoven C. Treatment of osteoarthritis with crystalline glucosamine sulfate. *MMW Fortschritte der Medizin* 2011;(153) Suppl 3:95-100.

2. Chainani-Wu N. Safety and anti-inflammatory activity of curcumin: a component of tumeric (Curcuma longa). *Journal of Alternative and Complementary Medicine* 2003;9(1):161-8.

3. Winther K. et al. A powder made from seeds and shells of a rose-hip subspecies (*Rosa canina*) reduces symptoms of knee and hip osteoarthritis: a randomized, double-blind, placebo-controlled clinical trial. *Scandinavian Journal of Rheumatology* 2005; 34(4):302-308.

4. Christensen R et al. Does the hip powder of *Rosa canina* (rosehip) reduce pain in osteoarthritis patients? – a meta-analysis of randomized controlled trials. *Osteoarthritis and Cartilage* 2008;(16):965-972.

5. Warholm O, Skaar S, Hedman E, Mřlmen HM, Eik L. The effects of a standardized herbal remedy made from a subtype of *Rosa canina* in patients with osteoarthritis: a double-blind, randomized, placebo-controlled clinical trial. *Current Therapeutic Research* 2003;64:21-31.

6.   Holford P. *Say No to Arthritis*, London: Piatkus, 2006.

7.   Chiu PR, Hu YC, Huang TC, Hsieh BS, Yeh JP, Cheng HL, Huang LW, Chang KL. Vitamin C protects chondrocytes against monosodium iodoacetate-induced osteoarthritis by multiple pathways. *International Journal of Molecular Science* 2016;18(1): pii-E38.

8.   Hung M, Bounsanga J, Voss MW, Gu Y, Crum AB, Tang P. Dietary and supplemental vitamin C and D on symptom severity and physical function in knee osteoarthritis. *Journal of Nutrition in Gerontology and Geriatrics* 2017;36(2-3):121-133.

9.   Thomas S, Browne H, Mobasheri A, Rayman MP. What is the evidence for a role for diet and nutrition in osteoarthritis? *Rheumatology (Oxford)* 2018; 57(Suppl 4): iv61–iv74.

10.   Chen HY, Cheng FC, Pan HC et al. Magnesium enhances exercise performance via increasing glucose availability in the blood, muscle, and brain during exercise. *PLoS One* 2014; 9(1).

11.   Randall C, Randall H, Dobbs F, Hutton C, Sanders H. Randomized controlled trial of nettle sting for treatment of base-of-thumb pain. *Journal Royal Society Medicine* 2000;93(6):305-9.

12.   Grover AK, Samson SE. Benefits of antioxidant supplements for knee osteoarthritis: rationale and reality. *Nutrition Journal* 2016;15:1.

13.   Knuesel O, Weber M, Suter A. *Arnica montana* gel in osteoarthritis of the knee: an open, multicenter clinical trial. *Advanced Therapeutics* 2002;19(5):209-18.

14.   Widrig R, Suter A, Saller R, Melzer J. Choosing between NSAID and arnica for topical treatment of hand osteoarthritis in a randomised, double-blind study. *Rheumatology International* 2007;27(6):585-91.

15.   Staiger C. Comfrey: A Clinical Overview. *Phytotherapy Research* 2012; 26(10): 1441–1448.

16.   La Porta C, Bura SA, Negrete R, Maldonado R. Involvement of the endocannabinoid system in osteoarthritis pain. *European Journal of Neuroscience* 2014;39(3):485-500.

17.   Chopra A, Lavin P, Patwardhan B, Chitre D. A 32-week randomized, placebo-controlled clinical evaluation of RA-11, an Ayurvedic drug, on osteoarthritis of the knees. *Journal of Clinical Rheumatology* 2014; (10):236.

Chapter 8: Therapies to manage pain

1. Vickers AJ, Cronin AM, Maschino AC, et al. Acupuncture for chronic pain: individual patient data meta-analysis. *Archives of Internal Medicine* 2012;172:1444-1453.

2. Corbett MS, Rice SJC, Madurasinghe V, et al. Acupuncture and other physical treatments for the relief of pain due to osteoarthritis of the knee: Network meta-analysis. *Osteoarthritis Cartilage* 2013;21:1290-1298.

Chapter 9: Practical ideas to make life easier

1. Wallace IJ, Worthington S, Felson DT, Jurmain RD, Wren KT, Maijanen H, Woods RJ, Lieberman DE. Knee osteoarthritis has doubled in prevalence since the mid-20th century. *Proceedings National Academy Science USA* 2017;114(35):9332-9336.

2. Health and Safety Executive. *Work-related ill health and occupational disease in Great Britain*. www.hse.gov.uk/statistics/causdis/ (accessed 24 June 2019).

3. *On Your Feet Britain*. www.onyourfeetday.com (accessed 24 June 2019).

4. Buckley JP, Hedge A, Yates T, Copeland RJ, Loosemore M, Hamer M, Bradley G, Dunstan DW. The sedentary office: an expert statement on the growing case for change towards better health and productivity. *British Journal of Sports Medicine* 2015;49:1357-1362.

Chapter 10: The power of sleep and the weather

1. Quoted in Feurstein, G. *Yoga Gems: A Treasury of Practical and Spiritual Wisdom from Ancient and Modern Masters*. Bantam. 2002.

2. Timmermans EJ, van der Pas S, Schaap LA, Sánchez-Martínez M, Zambon S, Peter R, Pedersen NL, Dennison EM, Denkinger M, Castell MV, Siviero P, Herbolsheimer F, Edwards MH, Otero A, Deeg DJ. Self-perceived weather sensitivity and joint pain in older people with osteoarthritis in six European countries: results from the European Project on OSteoArthritis (EPOSA). *BMC Musculoskeletal Disorders* 2014;15:66.

3. McAlindon T, Formica M, Schmid CH, Fletcher J. Changes in barometric pressure and ambient temperature influence osteoarthritis pain. *American Journal of Medicine* 2007;120(5):429-34.

4. Timmermans EJ, Schaap LA, Herbolsheimer F, Dennison EM, Maggi S, Pedersen NL, Castell MV, Denkinger MD, Edwards MH, Limongi F, Sánchez-Martínez M, Siviero P, Queipo R, Peter R, van der Pas S, Deeg DJ; EPOSA Research Group. The influence of weather conditions on joint pain in older people with osteoarthritis: Results from the European Project on OsteoArthritis (EPOSA). *Journal of Rheumatology* 2015;42(10):1885-92.

Chapter 11: Lonely, depressed and stressed

1. Age UK. *All the Lonely People, Loneliness in Later Life*. Age UK. 2018. www.ageuk.org.uk/latest-press/articles/2018/october/all-the-lonely-people-report/ (accessed 24 May 2019).

2. House JS, Landis KR, Umberson D. Social relationships and health. *Science* 1988; (241): 540–545.

3. Cleland S. Hidden impact: Arthritis and mental wellbeing. *Arthritis Care*. arthritiscare.org.uk/assets/000/001/731/Hidden_impact_report_-_web_ISSUE_2_original.pdf?1494240069 (accessed 25 June 2019).

Chapter 12: Soups, juices and meals with ginger and turmeric

1. Khanna D, Sethi G, Ahn KS, Pandey MK, Kunnumakkara AB, Sung B, Aggarwal A, Aggarwal BB. Natural products as a gold mine for arthritis treatment. *Current Opinion Pharmacology* 2007;7(3):344–351.

2. Kuptniratsaikul V1, Thanakhumtorn S, Chinswangwatanakul P, Wattanamongkonsil L, Thamlikitkul V. Efficacy and safety of Curcuma domestica extracts in patients with knee osteoarthritis. *Journal of Alternative & Complementary Medicine* 2009;15(8):891-897.

Index

Index